# Animal Experimentation
A Guide to the Issues, Third Edition

An essential book for all those who conduct animal-based research or are involved in education and training, as well as regulators, supporters and opponents alike. This fully updated third edition includes discussion of genetically altered animals and associated welfare and ethical issues that surround the breeding programmes in animal based research. The book discusses the origins of vivisection, the advances in human and non-human welfare made possible by animal experimentation, moral objections, and alternatives to the use of animals in research. It also examines the regulatory umbrella under which experiments are conducted in Europe, USA and Australasia. The author highlights the future responsibilities of researchers who will be working with animals, and offers practical advice on experimental design, literature search, consultation with colleagues, and the importance of the ongoing search for alternatives.

**Vaughan Monamy** is an associate professor of Science and Science Ethics at the Australian Catholic University in Sydney. He has provided expert advice to the Australian Government's Animal Welfare and Gene Technology Ethics Committees, and has been awarded an Australian Government Learning and Teaching Citation for outstanding contributions to university student learning.

'. . . a succinct, accessible and balanced introduction to the controversy surrounding the use of animals in scientific research, product testing and education. . . . The guide's coverage of relevant issues is international in scope . . . especially suited to students planning to begin careers in the biological sciences, including as researchers, veterinarians, teachers, regulators or administrators.'
*Martin Stephens, Center for Alternatives to Animal Testing, John Hopkins University*

'. . . a "must-read" for any student or scientist involved in animal experimentation at any level.'
*Michael Brands, The Physiologist*

'. . . a thoughtful consideration of both the pros and cons of animal research . . . an excellent guide to the issues [of which] current teachers of biology and biomedical science should take note.'
*Asif A. Ghazanfar, Animal Behaviour*

Vaughan Monamy

# Animal Experimentation

*A Guide to the Issues*

Third Edition

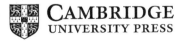

CAMBRIDGE
UNIVERSITY PRESS

# CAMBRIDGE
## UNIVERSITY PRESS

University Printing House, Cambridge CB2 8BS, United Kingdom

One Liberty Plaza, 20th Floor, New York, NY 10006, USA

477 Williamstown Road, Port Melbourne, VIC 3207, Australia

4843/24, 2nd Floor, Ansari Road, Daryaganj, Delhi – 110002, India

79 Anson Road, #06–04/06, Singapore 079906

Cambridge University Press is part of the University of Cambridge.

It furthers the University's mission by disseminating knowledge in the pursuit of education, learning, and research at the highest international levels of excellence.

www.cambridge.org
Information on this title: www.cambridge.org/9781107162020
10.1017/9781316678329

© Vaughan Monamy 2017
First edition © Cambridge University Press 2000

This publication is in copyright. Subject to statutory exception and to the provisions of relevant collective licensing agreements, no reproduction of any part may take place without the written permission of Cambridge University Press.

First published 2000
Second edition 2009
Third edition 2017

Printed in the United States of America by Sheridan Books, Inc., February 2017

*A catalogue record for this publication is available from the British Library.*

*Library of Congress Cataloging-in-Publication Data*
NAMES: Monamy, Vaughan, 1958– author.
TITLE: Animal experimentation : a guide to the issues / Dr. Vaughan Monamy.
DESCRIPTION: Third edition. | Cambridge ; New York, NY : Cambridge
    University Press, [2017] | Includes bibliographical references and index.
IDENTIFIERS: LCCN 2016040379| ISBN 9781107162020 (hardback : alk. paper) |
ISBN 9781316614945 (paperback)
SUBJECTS: LCSH: Animal experimentation. | Laboratory animals.
CLASSIFICATION: LCC HV4915 .M65 2017 | DDC 179/.4–dc23 LC record
    available at https://lccn.loc.gov/2016040379

ISBN 978-1-107-16202-0 Hardback
ISBN 978-1-316-61494-5 Paperback

Cambridge University Press has no responsibility for the persistence or accuracy of URLs for external or third-party Internet Web sites referred to in this publication and does not guarantee that any content on such Web sites is, or will remain, accurate or appropriate.

*We need another and a wiser and perhaps a more mystical concept of animals. . . . We patronize them for their incompleteness, for their tragic fate of having taken form so far below ourselves. And therein we err, and greatly err. For the animal shall not be measured by man. In a world older and more complete than ours they move finished and complete, gifted with extensions of the senses we have lost or never attained, living by voices we shall never hear. They are not brethren, they are not underlings; they are other nations, caught with ourselves in the net of life and time, fellow prisoners of the splendour and travail of the earth.*

Henry Beston (1928)

# Contents

## Preface to the third edition

In 2000, Cambridge University Press first published *Animal Experimentation: A Guide to the Issues*. A second edition was published in 2009. It is appropriate to reflect on what has happened since then in animal research, product testing and education within the accepted ethical framework of the 'three Rs' principles (Replacement, Reduction and Refinement: Russell and Burch 1959). What advances, for example, have been made in the search for alternatives to the use of vertebrates in biomedical research? Are there fewer animals used in research today? Or more? Has there been a continuation of the impetus to refine experimentation with animal welfare as the priority? Answering such questions requires a thorough reappraisal of where biomedicine, product testing and education are presently placing their emphases.

Twenty-first-century technological advances have resulted in an extraordinary increase in the number of procedures involving laboratory mice in genetic and molecular research. The enormous breeding programmes required to generate heterozygous strains of mice with genetic modifications has brought to bear entirely new welfare and ethical concerns regarding husbandry and 'surplus' animals. Are steps being taken in Britain, Europe, North America, China, South Korea, Brazil, Australasia and elsewhere to address these concerns? Were existing regulatory frameworks adequate, or have relevant statutes been necessarily updated?

In product and chemical safety testing, a trend towards fewer animals being used in toxicological screening is emerging in some countries. In Europe, there have been legislative changes that specifically prohibit newly animal-tested cosmetic products and ingredients being sold (European Commission 2009). In the United States, a toxicology vision document (National Research Council 2007) has urged the rapid adoption of cell-based assaying and other *in vitro* methods to replace *in vivo* testing. This has resulted in an acceleration in the uptake of *in vitro* and computer-based (*in silico*) methods with an associated reduction in laboratory animal use. Where else might such advances see a reduction in overall animal use?

Could discoveries in converging technologies such as interactive biotechnology, genome editing, synthetic biology and organ-on-a-chip biomimicry also point to a rapid replacement of animals in biological and medical research? Or will the technological advances that are making genetic alteration easier and less expensive result in a continued upsurge in animal use in experiments in these fields?

When *Animal Experimentation: A Guide to the Issues* was first written, general knowledge of computers and the internet was nowhere near as sophisticated as it is today. The acceptance of online applications such as 'Frog Dissection' as legitimate teaching tools has facilitated moves towards fewer classroom dissections. How widely has such smart device technology been adopted?

With such questions in mind, Cambridge University Press has published a completely updated third edition of *Animal Experimentation: A Guide to the Issues*. It is, once again, aimed at life science students, some of whom will follow careers as tomorrow's researchers, but at the same time its clarity of style and balanced treatment will enable lay people and experts to read it with equal ease. Students and researchers will find a non-intimidating, easy-to-read and readily understood introduction to the principal issues in the animal experimentation debate.

# Acknowledgements

The author is grateful for permission to reprint the following copyrighted material:

The frontispiece by Henry Beston, from *The Outermost House*. Copyright © 1928, 1949 © 1956 by Henry Beston. Copyright © 1977 by Elizabeth C. Beston. Reprinted by permission of Henry Holt and Co., Inc.

Quotation on p. 1 by Miriam Rothschild, from *Animals and Man. The Romanes Lecture for 1984–85* (Oxford: Clarendon Press, 1986). Reprinted by permission of Oxford University Press.

Quotation on p. 28 by Major Charles Hume, from *Man and Beast* (London: Universities Federation for Animal Welfare, 1962). Reprinted by permission of UFAW.

Quotations on p. 41 and pp. 53–54 by Albert Schweitzer from *Civilization and Ethics* third edition (London: Adam and Charles Black, 1955), *Indian Thought and Its Development* (London: Adam and Charles Black, 1936) and *My Life and Thought: An Autobiography* (London: Unwin Books, 1966). Reprinted by permission of Rhena Schweitzer Miller.

Quotations on p. 42–43 by Nicholas Humphrey, from R. Rodd, *Biology, Ethics and Animals* (Oxford: Clarendon Press, 1990), and Humphrey, N. K., *Consciousness Regained: Chapters in the Development of Mind* (Oxford: Oxford University Press, 1983). Reprinted by permission of Oxford University Press.

Quotation on p. 45 by Peter Singer, from *Practical Ethics*, third edition (Cambridge: Cambridge University Press, 2011). Reprinted with the permission of Peter Singer and Cambridge University Press.

Quotations on p. 46 by Peter Singer, from *Animal Liberation* second edition (New York: Thorston, 1990). Reprinted by permission of Blackwell Publishers, UK.

Quotation on pp. 46–47 by Tom Regan, from 'The case for animal rights', in P. Singer (ed.), *In Defense of Animals* (Oxford: Basil Blackwell, 1985). Reprinted by permission of Blackwell Publishers, UK.

Quotation on pp. 49–50 by Tom Regan, from 'The struggle for animal rights', in P. A. B. Clarke and A. Linzey (eds.), *Political Theory and Animal Rights* (1987; London: Pluto Press, 1990). Reprinted by permission of Pluto Press.

Quotations on p. 50 by Tom Regan, from *The Case for Animal Rights* (Berkeley: University of California Press, 1983). Reprinted by permission of University of California Press.

Quotations on p. 58, p. 61 and p. 97 by Smith, J. A. and Boyd, K. M. (eds.), from *Lives in the Balance: The Ethics of Using Animals in Biomedical Research* (Oxford: Oxford University Press, 1991). Reprinted by permission of Oxford University Press.

Quotation on p. 68 by Martin Walsh and Jon Richmond, from *School Science Review* 87(319): 85–89. Reprinted by permission of Jon Richmond.

Quotation on p. 78 by William Paton, from *Man and Mouse: Animals in Medical Research*, second edition (Oxford: Oxford University Press, 1993). Reprinted by permission of Oxford University Press.

Quotation on p. 102 by William Russell and Rex Burch, from *The Principles of Humane Experimental Technique* (London: Universities Federation for Animal Welfare, 1959/1992). Reprinted by permission of Cleo Paskal.

Issues in animal experimentation

> Looking back at the first half of my life as a zoologist I am particularly
> impressed by one fact: none of my teachers, lecturers, or professors with
> whom I came into contact ... none of the directors of laboratories where
> I worked, and none of my co-workers ever discussed with me, or each
> other in my presence, *the ethics of zoology*. No one ever suggested that
> one should respect the lives of animals in the laboratory or that they, and
> not the experiments, however fascinating and instructive, were worthy of
> greater consideration.
>
> *Miriam Rothschild (1986, p. 50)*

AIMS

The purpose of this book is to introduce life science students to the major issues that constitute modern debate about animal experimentation. Many such students will complete tertiary studies and go on to become the new generation of scientists. Those in the medical and allied health professions may only be exposed to animal experimentation in their undergraduate years. Others, such as geneticists, molecular biologists, veterinarians, physiologists, zoologists and agricultural scientists, may be actively involved in animal research at a postgraduate level and beyond. The welfare of animals in their care will continue to be of major concern to their employers, the granting bodies that fund their scientific research and to the public at large.

At some stage all such students will have to make a personal decision about the extent to which they are prepared to use research animals. Such decisions may influence potential career options. Most will be able to justify, to themselves and others, many forms of experimentation. Conversely, others will find that they are incapable of any intrusive procedure involving certain sentient animals. For some, sentience will not be an issue – they will be unable to experiment using *any* animals. I argue that decisions as serious as this ought to be taken only after informed discussion about major issues in animal experimentation.

These decisions will inevitably be made against a backdrop of differing societal and personal opinions about what is, and is not, appropriate treatment of animals. Adrian Franklin (2007) reported ambivalence and inconsistencies in the attitudes of people towards the treatment of animals in general. In his survey, almost all respondents (93 per cent) were comfortable with the idea of the humane killing of animals for food. But what happens if you muddy the waters a little? People have vastly different opinions about the treatment of particular species. In western society, it is acceptable to kill lambs for food but it is unacceptable to kill dogs for the same purpose. What about wildlife? In Australia there is ongoing debate about whether kangaroos that are killed in pastoral areas when numbers become too high ought to be used for food (Franklin 2007). Again, opinions differ and rational arguments in favour of kangaroo culling for human consumption do not necessarily gel with the emotional responses people may have when considering the eating of that nation's wildlife symbol.

Similarities are evident in any discussion of animal experimentation. Surveys of general attitudes to the use of animals for experimental and teaching purposes have consistently reported the majority of people in favour of such practices, where the procedures are important and suffering is minimised (e.g. Pifer, Shimizu and Pifer 1994; Franklin 2007; Leaman, Latter and Clemence 2014; Joffe et al. 2016). Another laboratory animal use, in product testing, does not receive the same level of public support. In response to the statement: 'It is acceptable to use animals in scientific research to test … chemicals that could harm people', Leaman, Latter and Clemence (2014) reported only 41 per cent of Britons in favour (pp. 15–16). In a comprehensive review of public attitudes towards animal based research, Ormandy and Schuppli (2014) also reported less support for animal use in product testing than in medical research.

Specific attitudes to laboratory animal use also differ by gender, nationality and how well informed are the survey respondents (Swami, Furnham and Christopher 2008; Leaman, Latter and Clemence 2014; Ormandy and Schuppli 2014). The species of animal used, too, can influence public attitudes (Crettaz von Roten 2012; Ormandy, Schuppli and Weary 2012).

Ultimately, though, most people who answer survey questions will never test potentially harmful chemicals on laboratory animals, nor will they perform any animal experiments. Many of the readers of this book will, and it is my contention that it is these people who need to be most informed. You must be able to determine what you are, and are not, capable of doing, and to express these opinions clearly and openly.

This book, therefore, aims to introduce to its readers important issues which have arisen out of the animal experimentation debate, which will assist them in making well-thought-out decisions. Not many students are fully conversant with the origins of modern animal experimentation practices, and fewer still with the intricacies of philosophical debate about the moral status of animals. In an increasing number of nations, animal experimentation is governed by legislation that aims to ensure that animals are used in ways in which suffering is minimised. It is important to know how the day-to-day practice of animal experimentation is regulated. Are you aware of the increasing number of available alternatives to using animals in experiments? By the time you have read this book, it is hoped that such information will assist you as you explore your thoughts and feelings about the use of research animals. You, too, have a voice in any discussion of animal experimentation.

Debate over issues in animal experimentation has come a long way, particularly since the 1970s. No longer does reasoned debate take the following form: opponent: 'All experimentation must cease!'; proponent: 'You're being totally sentimental; scientists know best!'. Instead (thankfully), contemporary discussions involve such issues as: What constitutes an essential experiment? What is appropriate conduct when using animals in research? What alternatives to using animals are available? In many countries (e.g. Australia, Canada and New Zealand), such debate is conducted against a background of progressive legislation that ensures, through a system of enforced self-regulation involving institutional ethics committees, that all experimentation, from undergraduate rat dissections to complex surgery on cats, dogs or wildlife, is reviewed and approved before such procedures take place. Other countries (e.g. Britain) rely on rigorous government regulation and a staff of inspectors rather than on self-regulation in addition to an ethical review process. Whatever the regulatory framework, its presence also acts to ensure that most public concerns about the unrestricted conduct of experiments are allayed.

Nevertheless, whenever an emotive issue is under discussion, opinions will differ. For those who are vehemently opposed to the use of animals for scientific research, no experiment will ever be considered essential, no conduct when using research animals will be deemed appropriate. At the other end of the spectrum there still may be advocates of scientific research free from any regulation. From this perspective, the welfare of human beings will always outweigh the welfare of non-human beings, and the quest for knowledge must never be hindered by what may be interpreted as ignorance or sentimentalism.

Wherever you or I choose to stand along this continuum, we must never lose sight of the fact that many of the medical benefits humanity carries with it in the twenty-first century arose through the use of research animals. Dreaded diseases such as poliomyelitis were once a scourge that ended many a young person's life. Survivors bore crippling limb deformities or were kept alive using artificial respirators. Because of experiments in which monkeys were integral, polio no longer poses the dire threat it did in the twentieth century. When a vaccine is developed which reduces the risk of humans becoming infected with human immunodeficiency virus (Gray *et al.* 2016; Harmon *et al.* 2016), it is certain that animals will have had a role to play in ensuring that such a treatment is safe for people to use.

So why is there a dilemma? Why do some students and researchers feel they are unable to conduct experiments involving certain animals? Why are scientists attacked, verbally and physically, for participating in research which may provide similar breakthroughs to that made in the containment of polio (Cressey 2011)? What is it that some sections of society find so reprehensible in such scientific activity? The answers to all such questions have an ethical basis. Few in society would object to an increased quality of life, human or non-human, for reasons other than ethical ones. For some, it is simply that the price of such advances may be too high. Thinking opponents of animal experimentation argue that for every experimental procedure that involves research animals, the means must justify the end. Radical opponents of animal experimentation argue (sometimes violently) that the end can never justify the means.

For people not involved in animal experimentation in any direct sense (remember, everybody who buys commercial products that have been tested on animals, or who has taken antibiotics or many other forms of medication is involved, indirectly), it is a relatively simple thing to be generally in favour of, or opposed to, research that involves animals. Most people are not working in laboratories, however. If you are to be part of the next generation of scientists, you might be. Readers have to determine what they are, and are not, capable of doing with research animals in their care. After all, if you are unable to justify aspects of your work to yourself, you will have difficulty justifying them to others.

What you will learn in your chosen field is that science demands professional objectivity from its adherents – little, if any, room is available for subjectivity, sentimentality and value judgements. Yet you, as scientists, are only human. You may find yourselves in the position of having to justify certain activities conducted within your laboratories which, if conducted outside them, might be viewed as barbaric. A provocative example: Why is it that a researcher can spend his or her weekend at home playing with a family pet and then, on Monday morning, return to their laboratory and test a potentially harmful chemical compound on stray or unwanted dogs? What is it about the donning of a white coat and the entering of the clinical atmosphere of a laboratory that can create an air of professional detachment? Opponents of animal experimentation may argue that such a scientist simply has ceased to feel. The scientists will argue that their work is of sufficient importance to the community at large to outweigh their feelings. Such scientists learn to manage the tension that arises between their professional objectivity and their personal feelings. For some readers, learning how to manage similar tensions will be an essential part of their education.

Contrary to what some opponents of animal experimentation may believe, it is both unfair and incorrect to state that western scientists currently conducting animal experiments are not fully conversant with their responsibilities. The overwhelming majority of practising scientists with whom I have been associated have a profound respect for the sacrifice made by their experimental subjects. They understand and work within their legal obligations and are in tune with the commonly voiced concerns of an increasingly well-informed general public. Modern society (rightly) insists that investigators increasingly pursue what are known as the 'three Rs' of modern research (Russell and Burch 1959). Namely:

- a *replacement* of animals in research, which follows on from an active development of alternatives;
- a *reduction* in the numbers of animals used in experiments;
- a *refinement* of laboratory and field techniques to reduce invasiveness and/or to increase the value of the results.

The 'three Rs' can be achieved in many ways. One tremendously important way is to alert science students to their future obligations as a part of their curriculum. In the European Union, appropriate training is now mandated (2010/63/EU Directive; Franco and Olsson 2014) and it should be an ideal of all modern nations that no university be able to graduate students from the biological or medical sciences who have not been educated formally in theories and practices that promote the humane care of animals used for scientific purposes. It is towards this goal that this book is directed.

### DEFINITIONS

For clarity, it is necessary to define certain terms that will be used throughout. *Animal* is used in its broadest sense to encompass all animate life forms. Where necessary, I will differentiate between human and non-human animals. Much discussion about animal experimentation is concerned only with certain 'higher' animals. Instead of using 'higher' to describe those animals with which we most associate (i.e. vertebrates generally and certain mammals in particular), I will refer to their *sentience*. A *sentient* animal not only has an awareness of its surroundings but is capable of suffering and experiencing pain. Pain is a difficult concept to define, and I deal with this in Chapter 7.

I use the term(s) *animal experiment(ation)* when discussing the use of live animals in research in the biological, ecological, psychological and medical technological sciences. The term also is appropriate to describe animal use in xenotransplantation and the generation of genetically altered and cloned animals, the production of biological extracts and the testing of consumer products, drugs and food. *Vivisection,* in the strictest sense, is the partial or complete dissection of live animals for research purposes. This is the definition that will be applied here. The word dates from a time when the majority of experiments involved dissection. *Anti-vivisection(ists)* is used to describe the stance of opposition (and its advocates) to this form of animal experimentation.

In many countries, research institutions now have committees that consider ethical aspects of research which involves sentient animals. They come under many names, so in this book, for consistency, all are referred to as *Animal Ethics Committees (AECs)*.

SCOPE

Currently, information on all aspects of animal welfare is available online and in many printed publications. Hundreds of articles have been written by moral philosophers, scientists and others advocating increased consideration for research animals. Many documents, too, are available that defend existing research procedures. In this book, I outline much of this extensive and specialised information for the readers for whom it is of the most value – the next generation of life scientists.

In the following chapters, readers will be introduced to the past, the present and the future of animal research.

- The origins of western vivisection are traced, and the parallel rise in opposition to such practices is discussed in context.
- Some of the many advances in human and non-human welfare that have been made possible by experiments which have involved research animals are described. Particular attention is given to the rapid growth in the number of animals bred and used in genetic alteration and associated research.

- The principal moral objections to animal experimentation are introduced and readers are urged to find an ethical position with which they are most comfortable.
- The regulatory umbrellas under which experiments are conducted in western countries are discussed.
- Efforts made towards finding alternatives to animal experimentation are given their full due.

By the time they reach the end of this book, readers should be in a better position to consider their responses to the complexities inherent in any discussion of animal experimentation. Numerous references are provided for those who wish to enquire more extensively into particular areas of interest. These are intended to be illustrative rather than exhaustive and you are encouraged to use them as a stepping stone to further reading.

A history of animal experimentation

> Those who think that science is ethically neutral confuse the findings of
> science, which are, with the activity of science, which is not.
>
> *Jacob Bronowski (1956, pp. 63–64)*

## THE ORIGINS OF VIVISECTION IN EUROPE

Early records of vivisection procedures provide sobering reading. However, it is worthwhile to examine some of them in order to understand how public concern over animal experimentation arose. We also need to consider the origins of western scientific practices and the prevailing societal attitudes towards them. Readers interested in a complete history of animal experimentation and further insight into the historically important attitudes of humans towards animals are referred to excellent discussions elsewhere (Maehle and Tröhler 1987; Rupke 1987; French 1999; Ryder 2000; Franco 2013).

Live animals, both human and non-human, appear to have been first used in ancient times, principally to satisfy anatomical curiosity. In the third century BC, the Alexandrian physicians Herophilus and Erisistratus are recorded as having examined functional differences between sensory nerves, motor nerves and tendons (Singer 1957). Galen of Pergamum (AD 129–199), a Greek physician working in Rome, catalogued these early experiments, as well as conducting his own. He described, for the first time, the complexities of the cardiopulmonary system, and speculated on brain and spinal cord function (Duckworth, Lyons and Towers 1962). All such procedures were conducted without anaesthetics (which were not discovered until the mid-nineteenth century), and it is interesting to note the expression of his feelings during such experiments. When investigating the anatomy of the brain, Galen preferred to vivisect pigs to 'avoid seeing the unpleasant expression of the ape' (Maehle and Tröhler 1987, p. 15). Galen

(1956) left a legacy for future scientists. In *De Anatomicis Administratio-nibus* (On Anatomical Procedures), he detailed precise experimental methods and indicated which instruments would be best to perform many specific procedures.

Documentation of vivisection from the Dark Ages is scanty. It was not until Galen's records were rediscovered during the sixteenth century that there appears to have been any renewal of interest in anatomy and scientific methods. Such experiments often were conducted as public demonstrations. Belgian Andreas Vesalius (1514–1564) and his students in Padua, Italy, illustrated public lectures on anatomy by using systematic non-human vivisection. An animal, usually a dog, would be cut open while still alive and the function of each organ would be speculated upon as it was located. It appears, from the records of these procedures, that the welfare of their experimental subjects was a low priority for these early vivisectionists. Maehle and Tröhler (1987) recorded that the experiments of one of Vesalius' pupils, Realdo Colombo (1516–1559), involving pregnant dogs, were greatly admired by members of the Catholic clergy:

> Colombo pulled a foetus out of the dog's womb and, hurting the young in front of the bitch's eyes, he provoked the latter's furious barking. But as soon as he held the puppy to the bitch's mouth, the dog started licking it tenderly, being obviously more concerned about the pain of its offspring than about its own suffering. When something other than the puppy was held in front of its mouth, the bitch snapped at it in a rage. The clergymen expressed their pleasure in observing this striking example of motherly love even in the 'brute creation' (cited in Maehle and Tröhler 1987, p. 18).

PREVAILING HUMANIST ATTITUDES TO ANIMALS

### The Christian view

It may be difficult for readers to understand the apparent indifference to suffering exhibited in southern Europe at this time. What must be considered, however, is that the Christian church subscribed to the view that humans, blessed with the divine gift of reason, did not share a common evolutionary lineage with other animals. Three hundred years earlier, St. Thomas Aquinas (1225–1274) had declared in his *Summa Theologiae* (1260) that humans were unique; all other animals were incapable of rationality because they possessed no mind. Only humans had a soul and the power to reason. Without a soul, animals were merely objects, devoid of personality or rights. They existed only for human needs and were bereft of moral status (Linzey and Clarke 2004). This is not to say that the Christian church supported a view that an absence of moral status meant that any form of cruelty was acceptable. The church recognised that the animals over which humans had been given dominion were a part of God's creation and, for that reason, were worthy of respect. Many animals, such as the dove, were symbolised as a part of Christian worship, and St. Francis of Assisi (1181–1226) was venerated because of his sympathetic attitude towards animals. At the same time, however, Christian society did not see the infliction of pain on animals (or humans, for that matter) as objectionable in itself if it was an unintended consequence of some 'higher' purpose. However, the gratuitous infliction of pain was viewed as morally reprehensible cruelty. The inescapable suffering of animals during experimental procedures, such as that described above, was not seen in any way as cruel while it was conducted in the pursuit of greater knowledge.

### Descartes and the influence of Cartesian thought

The seventeenth century saw an explosion of interest in scientific activity. British Lord Chancellor Francis Bacon (1561–1626) sustained the Christian anthropocentric (human-centred) view in his *De Augmentis Scientarium* (The Advancement of Learning, Bacon (1605) 2001). He asserted that much could be learned of the human body and its workings by vivisecting animals and that such dissection obviated the need for the morally repugnant (but nonetheless fairly common) practice of human vivisection involving criminals.

French philosopher René Descartes (1596–1650) was to play an important role in early debate over vivisection. Christian-centred humanist attitudes, so prevalent throughout Europe, became exaggerated into a mechanistic philosophy following the publication of Descartes' *Discours de la Méthode* ((1637) 1984). Here, Descartes stated that it was possible to describe humans and other animals as complex machines: their bodies would obey known laws of mechanics. Descartes also believed, however, that the divine gift of the soul distinguished the human animal from all others. Only humans were conscious and capable of rational thought. Only humans were capable of acts of free will, and had true language. Only humans could declare *Cogito ergo sum* – 'I think therefore I am'. The reactions of animals were dismissed as mere reflex, the response of automata (Rosenfield 1940). This concept of 'beast-machine' was critical to the way in which scientists viewed animals. It provided a convenient ideology for early vivisectionists: How could animals suffer real pain if they had no soul? How could animals suffer real pain if they had no real consciousness? In Descartes' writings was found a reason to discount the behavioural responses of animals to vivisection (which would be described as symptomatic of pain in humans) as the mere mechanical reactions of robots. Cries of pain in animals were now interpreted as the squeaking of unoiled cogs. (Note, however, that John Cottingham (1978) has argued for a reappraisal of the 'monstrous' Cartesian thesis. He believed that Descartes had been mis-interpreted as denying *all* consciousness to animals. A response to this argument has been offered by Tom Regan (1983) pp. 3–9.)

### THE RISE OF MODERN BIOMEDICAL STUDIES

In a series of formative experiments conducted at the anatomy school in Padua in 1628, Briton William Harvey (1578–1657) demonstrated the circulation of blood using animals, extrapolated the discovery to humans and in so doing showed the value of vivisection not only for satisfying anatomical curiosity but also for comparative physiological investigation (Harvey (1628) 1978). Questions long pondered about how we breathe, digest food and so on suddenly appeared to have physio-logical answers. As a result of Harvey's experiments, many other scien-tific investigators were eager to delve into the workings of the animal body. The rate of animal experimentation increased – an increase that was to continue beyond the seventeenth and into the eighteenth and nineteenth centuries.

Frenchman François Magendie (1783–1855) was among the first to determine that many bodily processes resulted from the co-functioning of several organs. This realisation set in motion numerous experiments that involved manipulative procedures rather than just internal observations. Although many of his experiments were 'hit-or-miss', Magendie is described as the founder of modern physiology (Ryder 2000).

Another landmark in physiology came with the publication of *Introduction à l'étude de la médicine expérimentale* ((1865) 1957) by one of Magendie's students, Claude Bernard (1813–1878). In this work, Bernard declared that a precise approach to experimentation must involve the study of one parameter while holding extraneous variables constant (this remains as a fundamental approach in modern science). In addition, he responded to a growing number of critics of vivisection by offering a powerful philosophical rationale for experimental medicine. Bernard ((1865) 1957) posed:

> Have we the right to make experiments on animals and vivisect them? . . . I think we have this right, wholly and absolutely. It would be strange indeed if we recognised man's right to make use of animals in every walk of life, for domestic service, for food, and then forbade him to make use of them for his own instruction in one of the sciences most useful to humanity. No hesitation is possible; the science of life can be established only through experiment, and we can save living beings from death only after sacrificing others. Experiments must be made either on man or on animals. Now I think that physicians already make too many dangerous experiments on man, before carefully studying them on animals. I do not admit that it is moral to try more or less dangerous or active remedies on patients in hospitals, without first experimenting with them on dogs; for I shall prove . . . that results obtained on animals may all be conclusive for man when we know how to experiment properly. (Bernard (1865) 1957, pp. 102–103)

The work of physiologists such as Magendie and Bernard, coupled with the discovery of the anaesthetic properties of ether (by Crawford Long in 1842, and by William Morton in 1847), resulted in an adoption of technically sophisticated surgical procedures. Animal experimentation became routine in an increasing number of physiology laboratories throughout Europe. In Britain, the 1876 *Cruelty to Animals Act* (see Chapter 3) required meticulous registration of the numbers of research animals used in experiments each year. These records show that the number of procedures involving research animals increased from 311 in 1880 to over 95 000 in 1910.

The end of the nineteenth century saw vast improvements in aseptic surgical techniques and the development of bacteriology and immunology. Key medical breakthroughs, such as the discovery, in 1882, of the bacterium responsible for tuberculosis, and of a diphtheria antitoxin in 1894 (which rapidly reduced infant mortality from 40 per cent to 10 per cent in those afflicted), led to broad public acceptance of animal experimentation (Turner 1980).

More medical breakthroughs occurred at the beginning of the twentieth century, further emphasising the value of using animals in biomedical research. These included: the extraction of the first hormone (1902); a chemical treatment for syphilis (1909: French 1999); and the isolation of insulin in the 1920s by Banting and Best (White 2014), leading to the development of an effective treatment of diabetes mellitus (Bliss 1982). Such spectacular advances attracted enormous public acclaim and heralded the modern era of animal experimentation. In Britain, the numbers of animals used in experiments increased to exceed 1 million per year in 1945 and approach 6 million per year by 1970 (UK Home Office 2016). Numbers had declined to 3 million by 1991 and were down to 2.7 million in 1998 (UK Home Office 2016). From 1995 until 2013, procedures other than those involved in the production of genetically altered animals continued this decline. UK Home Office (2014a) statistics show a 16 per cent reduction in procedures in that time.

However, an extraordinary increase in experimentation involving genetically altered animals increased total animal use to approach levels only really seen in the 1970s. From 1995, the number of procedures that commenced involving genetically altered animals rose from 12 per cent (of 2.8 million) to involve half of the 4.14 million procedures completed in 2015 (UK Home Office 2016, p. 9).[1]

[1] An amendment to the UK Animals (Scientific Procedures) Act (1986) to comply with European Union Directive 2010/63/EU (European Commission 2010) came into effect on 1 January 2013. Statistical data collection changed to reflect procedures *completed* rather than *initiated*. Direct comparisons of UK 2015 animal use statistics with earlier data should be made with caution (UK Home Office 2016, p. 7).

Animal use in the 15 countries that have been part the European Union since 1995 has been constant at approximately 11 million per year (European Commission 2013), but in countries such as Germany, animal numbers have risen due to the increase in the number of procedures involving genetically altered animals (Daneshian *et al.* 2015).

Increased government financial support led to the important improvements in preventative medicine and surgical techniques that today permit many to enjoy longer and enhanced lives. In 1989, the American Medical Association's Council on Scientific Affairs published an impressive list of medical advances made possible through research using animals. It included studies of anaesthesia, autoimmune deficiency syndrome (AIDS) and autoimmune diseases, behaviour, cardiovascular disease, cholera, diabetes, gastrointestinal surgery, genetics, haemophilia, hepatitis, infant health, infection, malaria, muscular dystrophy, nutrition, ophthalmology, organ transplantation, Parkinson's disease, prevention of rabies, radiobiology, reproductive biology, shock, the skeletal system and treatment of spinal injuries, toxoplasmosis, yellow fever and virology. Such research has resulted in enormous gains in human knowledge with subsequent benefits for human and non-human health.

This is an important point that deserves emphasis. We live in an unprecedented age where life-threatening illnesses are kept at bay to an extraordinary degree. Having lived all of our lives at such a time, it is easy to forget that as recently as 70 years ago many diseases, such as polio and tuberculosis, were common killers in our society. In early Victorian Britain, life expectancy at birth was 42 years. Today, life expectancy at birth in Britain (and all western nations) exceeds 80 years (World Health Organisation 2015). One important reason for this increase in longevity (without detracting from, for example, the role of enhanced public health measures, clean water and occupational safety laws) is the benefits that have stemmed from animal experimentation.

Given such a track record, how could anyone condemn such practices? Surely increases in human health standards, as well as increased productivity of domestic livestock or increased conservation outcomes for endangered species of wild animals through ecological investigations etc., outweigh any suffering involved in obtaining these advances?

This is at the heart of the matter. Some see that all experimentation is vital, ultimately beneficial and must be allowed to continue unchecked. At the other end of the spectrum are individuals who hold deep convictions that all animal experimentation is an abuse of other species for selfish human gain. If you choose a sub-set of humanity (say, the readers of this book) and quiz them on their personal attitudes, all will opt for a position somewhere along this continuum. Where you choose to stand will depend on many things, including career aspirations, vested interests, level of understanding of complex issues, personal moral views, religious beliefs and levels of compassion for certain animals. In the next chapter, readers are shown how objections to some animal experiments gained popular support, and why scientists increasingly had to defend particular experiments as essential before they were permitted to proceed.

Opposition to animal experimentation

How absurd, ... to say that beasts are machines, devoid of knowledge
and feeling, which perform all their operations in the same manner,
which learn nothing, which perfect nothing, etc! ... Barbarians seize
this dog, which surpasses man so greatly in his capacity for friendship;
they nail him to a table, and dissect him alive to show you the mesenteric
veins. You discover in him the same organs of feeling that are in
yourself. Answer me, machinist, has nature arranged all the springs of
feeling in this animal in order that he should not feel? Has he nerves in
order to be unmoved? Do not suppose such a pointless contradiction
in nature.

*Voltaire ((1764) 1962, pp. 112–113)*

INTRODUCTION

Opposition to the use of animals for research purposes is not an entirely
modern phenomenon. As the number of experiments had increased
over time, so too had resistance to them. In many countries, rigid
controls are now in force to prevent ill-considered exploitation of laboratory animals (see Chapter 6). These regulations had their origins in
nineteenth-century Britain, where opposition to painful animal experiments culminated in far-reaching legislation. The 1876 *Cruelty to
Animals Act* ensured for the first time that the welfare of laboratory
animals was a legitimate consideration. It is of value to examine the
reasons for the enabling of such legislation, and much of the ensuing
discussion is derived from the British experience.

EARLY OPPOSITION

The first people to record their uneasiness with respect to vivisection
were some professional physiologists. Only later did the general public
become passionately involved. Professional opposition was based on a
moral objection to perceived cruelty (remember, efficient anaesthesia was
not available until the mid-nineteenth century). In addition, questions

regarding the value of results gained from dying animals needed to be answered. Surely, 'the miserable torture of vivisection places the body in an unnatural state' (O'Meara 1655, cited in Maehle and Tröhler 1987, p. 22).

Experimental physiologists Robert Boyle (1627–1691), Robert Hooke (1635–1703) and Richard Lower (1631–1691) exhibited genuine concern for the welfare of some of their experimental subjects. Boyle had gained general popularity during the mid-seventeenth century after he used his 'pneumatick engine' to demonstrate publicly the effects on kittens of being placed in a vacuum (Franco 2013). Boyle spoke of excluding a kitten that had survived one air pump experiment from further trials because 'it was too severe to make him undergo the same measure again' (Shugg 1968a, p. 237). Hooke, after opening the thoracic cavity of a dog and observing the functioning of the animal's heart and lungs after the diaphragm had been cut away, kept the animal alive for over an hour by means of artificial respiration (a pipe inserted into its throat). In correspondence to Boyle, he confessed that he would be unable to repeat the procedure 'because it was cruel' (cited in Maehle and Tröhler 1987, p. 23). Richard Lower, also in correspondence to Boyle, drew attention to the tragedy of a donor dog's death during a blood transfusion experiment. At the same time, however, such men remained convinced that the costs in terms of the suffering of their experimental subjects were far outweighed by the potential, though unstated, benefits for humanity.

For the most part, early public opposition to vivisection was not based on a perception of cruelty. Rather, opposition was based on the argument that because of the fundamental differences (both anatomical and spiritual) believed to separate humans from other animals, little relevant benefit could be derived from experimentation on 'lesser' beings. Prevailing philosophical and religious views still regarded humans as completely different from other animals. Consequently, information gained by way of non-human vivisection could not legitimately be extrapolated to the human form.

By the eighteenth century, criticism of vivisection had become more widespread, but was still not a popular issue. Indignation was limited 'to scattered literati and the occasional humanitarian pamphleteer'

(French 1975, p. 17). Perhaps for the first time, critics were questioning what was appropriate human behaviour towards non-humans. For example, in the last year of his life, poet Alexander Pope (1688–1744) became a committed anti-vivisectionist after witnessing the blood circulation experiments of Reverend Stephen Hales (1677–1761):

> he commits most of these barbarities with the thought of its being of use to man; but how do we know that we have a right to kill creatures that we are so little above as dogs, for our curiosity, or even for some use to us? (cited in French 1975, p. 16)

Pope was not alone. Samuel Johnson (1709–1784) fiercely attacked vivisectionists through his weekly newspaper, *The Idler*:

> Among the inferior Professors of medical knowledge is a race of wretches, whose lives are only varied by varieties of cruelty ... What is alleged in defense of these hateful practices everyone knows, but the truth is, that by knives, fire, and poison knowledge is not always sought and is very seldom attained. The experiments that have been tried are tried again ... I know not that by living dissections any discovery has been made by which a single malady is more easily cured. And if knowledge of physiology has been somewhat increased, he surely buys knowledge dear, who learns the use of the lacteals at the expense of his humanity. It is time that universal resentment should arise against these horrid operations, which tend to harden the heart, extinguish those sensations which give man confidence in man, and make physicians more dreadful than gout or stone. (cited in French 1975, pp. 16–17)

## UTILITARIANISM AND THE RISE OF POPULAR CONCERN

A platform of opposition to vivisection was being constructed, consisting of three central planks. First, surely non-human animals were, at best, only questionable models of the human condition. If so, why were scientists so keen to use them? Second, eighteenth-century English essayists and poets were rejecting Descartes' 'beast-machine' concept and were arguing that animals may well feel pain, and that this pain ought to be taken into consideration (Shugg 1968b). Third, and importantly, because anti-vivisectionists felt empathy with certain animals, compassionate people were looking for a philosophy that incorporated their concern for non-humans, arguing that animals ought to be afforded some form of moral status. Many sought to occupy this ethical dais, and argument was passionate and persuasive. The predominant doctrines of Cartesian and Thomist (after St. Thomas Aquinas) humanism were increasingly challenged by the new philosophy of *utilitarianism*. This creed professed that the only 'good' was pleasure and the only 'evil' was pain. To be a utilitarian meant that one should act to produce the greatest balance of pleasure over pain. The thoughts of philosopher Jeremy Bentham (1748–1832) played a central role in ensuing debate. He defined utility as

> that property in any object, whereby it tends to produce benefit, advantage, pleasure, good, or happiness, ... or ... to prevent the happening of mischief, pain, evil, or unhappiness to the party whose interest is considered. (Bentham (1789) 1970, pp. 11–12)

Did not a belief that animals were capable of feeling both pleasure and pain mean that they warranted similar consideration to humans? In *An Introduction to the Principles and Morals of Legislation* ((1789) 1970), Bentham emphasised that all humans were worthy of equal and humane consideration. As a footnote to this declaration he also suggested that a time may come when animals would also be afforded similar consideration:

> The day *may* come when the rest of the animal creation may acquire those rights which never could have been withholden from them but by the hand of tyranny. The French have already discovered that the blackness of the skin is no reason why a human being should be abandoned without redress to the caprice of a tormentor. It may one day come to be recognised that the number of the legs, the villosity of the skin, or the termination of the *os sacrum* are reasons equally insufficient for abandoning a sensitive being to the same fate. What else is it that should trace the insuperable line? Is it the faculty of reason, or perhaps the faculty of discourse? But a full-grown horse or dog is beyond comparison a more rational, as well as a more conversable animal, than an infant of a day or a week or even a month, old. But suppose they were otherwise, what would it avail? The question is not, Can they *reason*? nor Can they *talk*? but, Can they *suffer*? (Bentham (1789) 1970, p. 283: Bentham's italics)

Bentham was writing at a time when the French were beginning to oppose the capture and enslavement of Africans for labour in Europe and North America. It seemed only logical to him (but not to many of his contemporaries) that a similar ethical consideration ought to be extended beyond the human moral sphere to certain animals. This was an issue that was to feature prominently in the development of anti-vivisection organisations in England in the 1800s.

An earlier, but less well-known, challenge to humanism came in 1776 when Humphry Primatt published his *Dissertation on the Duty of Mercy and the Sin of Cruelty to Brute Animals*. Here, Primatt extended the principle of justice beyond the sphere of humans, to include all animals:

> Now, if amongst men, the difference of their powers of the mind, of their complexion, stature, and accidents of fortune, do not give any one man a right to abuse or insult any other man on account of these differences; for the same reason, a man can have no natural right to abuse or torment a beast, merely because a beast has not the mental powers of a man. (cited in Linzey 1989, pp. 32–33)

Primatt further insisted that

> superiority of rank or station may give ability to communicate happiness ... but it can give no right to inflict unnecessary or unmerited pain. (cited in Linzey 1989, p. 33)

The anthropocentric world view was being challenged by a more holistic notion that animals ought to be protected for their own sake. Whether an animal had a soul or not was no longer an issue – Primatt and Bentham had replaced it with a new criterion: *an animal's capacity to suffer*.

## REVOLUTION DURING THE NINETEENTH CENTURY

At the beginning of the nineteenth century, animal anti-cruelty societies had been concerned almost exclusively with the abolition of the essentially working-class pursuits of cock fighting and dog fighting, as well as horse baiting and bull baiting. Membership in animal welfare societies was reserved for the middle and upper classes (who, apparently, saw nothing wrong with their own hunting sports (Rupke 1987)). While institutionalised animal experimentation continued to be a greater-European phenomenon, few in Britain appeared concerned about its practice.

This attitude was to change following a scientific controversy that pitted the methods of an English anatomist, Sir Charles Bell (1774–1842), against those of the French physiologist, François Magendie. Following public lectures in London in 1824, Magendie was accused of unnecessary cruelty in experimentation (Cranefield 1974). It is not certain whether the fact that one scientist was French and the other English created the controversy, but his actions provoked the following response from the editor of the *London Medical Gazette* in 1829:

> We recollect, some years ago, a violent clamour was raised against the practice of experimenting upon living animals ... Certain lecturers were represented in the most odious light as unnecessarily torturing and sacrificing the lives of rabbits, frogs, dogs, and cats. The attention of the Parliament was called to the subject; the infliction of pains and penalties was threatened; and conviction, under a special statute, was, with difficulty, evaded. The appalling experiments of Magendie were the topic of the day; and ... correspondence ... excited a strong sensation. (cited in French 1975, p. 20)

Physiology as a scientific discipline was responding to a growing insistence on consideration for the welfare of research animals. In England, a contemporary of François Magendie, neurologist and physiologist Marshall Hall (1790–1857), pioneered welfare issues from within science. As early as 1831, he proposed that physiological procedures be regulated in a way that took into consideration the suffering of animals (Paton 1993). Hall believed that five specific rules should be applied to all experiments. A researcher who adhered to these rules would be in a strong position to resist any public imputations of cruelty. As a first requirement, no experiment was to take place if the necessary information could be gained by observation alone. Second, only experiments that would result in the fulfilment of clearly defined and *attainable* aims ought to proceed. Third, unnecessary repetition of experiments must be avoided – particularly if reputable physiologists had been responsible for the original experiments. (Hall was later to call for the formation of a professional society of English physiologists with a journal to record all experiments and to keep members informed of current procedures

(French 1975).) Fourth, all experiments must be conducted with a minimum of suffering. Finally, Hall proposed that all physiological experiments be witnessed by peers, further reducing the need for repetition.

Hall's far-reaching suggestions reflected an increasing societal abhorrence of animal cruelty, including painful vivisection. The Society for the Prevention of Cruelty to Animals (SPCA) had been inaugurated in 1824 and its members committed themselves to the principles of kindness to animals, educating the general public about cruelty, and to lobbying parliamentarians for the enactment of anti-cruelty legislation. Its objections to vivisection, however, were mild at first, and it maintained that some experiments were justifiable if conducted humanely. The SPCA received the patronage of Princess Victoria in 1835, and in 1840, as Queen Victoria, she gave permission for the society to use the 'Royal' prefix. Following the publication of evidence of the anaesthetic properties of ether in 1847, the RSPCA opposed all painful vivisection (French 1975). Throughout the nineteenth century, the RSPCA lobbied successfully for numerous changes to legislation. For example, the *Martins Act* (1822) was amended in 1835 to outlaw animal baiting; in 1854, dog-drawn carts were made illegal; and in 1869, game birds were accorded limited protection (Ryder 2000).

### The 1870s, and the UK Cruelty to Animals Act (1876)

In June 1874, Queen Victoria expressed her concern over the treatment of animals used in experiments in correspondence accompanying a private donation to the RSPCA (Ryder 2000). This royal interest coincided with wide-scale English public opposition in the 1870s. The British Association for the Advancement of Science was under tremendous pressure to be accountable publicly for the behaviour of its members. The association had already published guidelines in 1871 that aimed to minimise suffering and discourage conducting experiments which were of dubious scientific merit (Phillips and Sechzer 1989):

- No procedure which could be performed with anaesthesia should be done without it.
- No painful experiment was justifiable if it were only being conducted to illustrate an already known fact.

- Whenever painful experiments were necessary, every effort ought to be made to ensure the success of the procedure, so that the experiment need not be repeated. For this reason, no such experiments should be performed by unqualified scientists with insufficient instruments or assistance, or in places not suited to the purpose.
- Operations should not be performed using living animals merely for the purpose of gaining new operative skills.

English society had been rocked to its foundations a few years earlier by the publication of Charles Darwin's *On the Origin of Species by Natural Selection* ((1859) 2009). Darwin had provoked furious debate with his theory that human and non-human beings had a common ancestor. In 1871, he addressed the specific issue of human origins in *The Descent of Man, and Selection in Relation to Sex* ((1871) 2004). He was convinced that his theory of natural selection must apply to all animals and that humans could not be excluded. In so thinking, he rejected the idea that humans were designed by God to stand apart from the rest of creation. Such an idea flew in the face of contemporary Christian theology, undermining arguments that all non-humans were a gift from God, to be used by humanity to their own ends. One such end was, of course, scientific curiosity – but, if we were related to the animals, argued opponents of vivisection, how could we use them in experiments perceived as cruel? (Darwin himself steadfastly supported the advancement of science through experimentation but was utterly opposed to any form of cruelty.) Science in general, and biological science in particular, was in the public spotlight as never before.

On 4 May 1875, a Bill aimed at regulating vivisection was presented in the House of Lords. Eight days later, a contrary Bill allowing for a regulation-free experimental environment was introduced into the House of Commons (Ryder 2000). Because of the contradictory nature of the two Bills and an increasing public clamour, British Prime Minister Benjamin Disraeli appointed a Royal Commission of Inquiry to investigate laboratory procedures involving animals. It reported back to parliament in the following year. Briefly, it found no specific instances of laboratory animal abuse in the United Kingdom but did recommend that, for the first time, animal experimentation be regulated (French 1978). The House of Commons set about preparing appropriate legislation to this end.

In response, a lobby group, the Victoria Street Society for the Protection of Animals from Vivisection, had been formed by Frances Power Cobbe (1822–1904) to argue for the legal restriction of vivisection. The Victoria Street Society (as it became known) attracted enormous support. The most prominent members were clergymen, such as the Archbishops of Westminster and York and the Bishops of Oxford and Carlisle. Other members came from the judiciary and parliament, including the Lord Chief Justice Coleridge and the Earl of Shaftsbury. The poets Alfred, Lord Tennyson and Robert Browning also were powerful lobbyists for the protection of laboratory animals.

Cobbe and others argued, among other things, that anaesthesia must be a compulsory component of all animal experiments involving surgery, and that animals should be euthanased without recovering from the anaesthetic (French 1975). The Victoria Street Society maintained that legislation also was required to prohibit the use of cats, dogs or horses for vivisection. A Bill was drafted along these lines, the *Cruelty to Animals Act*, and introduced to the House of Lords in May 1876 for debate. However, scientists were far from satisfied and, forming a lobby group of their own, argued for compromise in the area of anaesthesia. It was argued that, in some cases, the use of anaesthesia could adversely affect results; others argued for the necessity of recovery of experimental subjects in certain procedures. Many claimed the right to use any animal species for any purpose. Such lobbying proved successful, and additional clauses were included in the draft legislation to permit such practices, where appropriate. Lobbying of individual parliamentarians by members of the Victoria Street Society and the RSPCA on one side and members of the General Medical Council on the other continued until August 1876, when the Bill received royal assent. In essence, the *Cruelty to Animals Act* (1876) required that any person wishing to perform experiments using live vertebrates must first be licensed, and all experiments involving cats, dogs, horses, mules and asses, or those conducted to illustrate lectures, be certified by the British Home Secretary.

The Victoria Street Society was disappointed with what they perceived as inadequate legislation and in 1878 changed their name (and aims) from 'the Protection of Animals from Vivisection' to the Victoria Street Society for the Abolition of Vivisection (French 1978). Eminent clergymen, such as the Archbishop of Westminster, Cardinal Manning (1808–1892), argued strongly for this cause:

> at the present day we are under the tyranny of the word Science. I believe in science most profoundly, within its own limits; but it has its own limits, and, when the word science is applied to matter which is beyond those limits, I don't believe in it, and as I believe that vivisection is susceptible of such excessive abuse – such facile abuse – such clandestine abuse – all over the land, and by all manner of people, I shall do all I can to restrain it to the utmost of my power. (Manning (1887) 1934, p. 11)

Abolition remained the goal of the Victoria Street Society until 1898 when internal divisions resulted in a more moderate line being taken by the renamed National Anti-Vivisection Society. Frances Cobbe resigned in protest and formed a new society, the rigidly abolitionist British Union for the Abolition of Vivisection. This society also had its champions, for example George Bernard Shaw:

> But I always regard a vivisector as a moral imbecile, and an intellectual imbecile. Consequently, I have a sort of benevolent feeling toward him, and I do not look upon him as an altogether grown-up and responsible person. (Shaw 1912, p. 2)

Public campaigning towards the abolition of vivisection continued to be frequent and intensive. Anti-vivisection societies were considered fashionable by many of Britain's élite. Consequently, the use of animals for scientific purposes was never far from public scrutiny. Richard Ryder (2000) illustrated this depth of feeling. He described the erection, in 1906 in Battersea Park, London, of a bronze statue in tribute to a dog used in experiments by staff and students at University College, London. The National Anti-Vivisection Society, with the approval of the Battersea Borough Council, included a plaque that bore the following inscription:

> In memory of the brown Terrier Dog done to death in the laborator-
> ies of University College in February 1903 after having endured
> vivisection extending over more than two months and having been
> handed over from one vivisector to another till death came to his
> release. Also in memory of the 232 dogs vivisected in the same place
> during the year 1902. Men and women of England: How long shall
> these things be? (cited in Ryder 2000, pp. 135–136)

In 1907, the statue was damaged by protesting medical students
from University College, London. They insisted that the statue and
inscription be removed. The council refused. The demonstrations
that ensued were violent and uncontrolled. On 10 December 1907,
about 100 medical students attempted to remove the memorial by
force and were opposed throughout the afternoon and into the night
by a large number of concerned citizens who wished to see the statue
remain as and where it was. Mounted police were called in to keep
the peace, arresting ten protesters in the process. In the weeks that
followed, medical students were joined by veterinary students in pro-
vivisection protest marches, and ultimately, a contingent of over
100 policemen had to be detailed to protect the statue from further
attacks (Ryder 2000).

Two years later the statue disappeared and, to date, has never been
found. A meeting called to protest its disappearance attracted several
thousand demonstrators to Trafalgar Square, London. As a martyr,
the brown dog had focussed the attention of the public on what
was considered unnecessary cruelty conducted under the auspices
of science.

Continuous lobbying resulted in the Second Royal Commission of
Vivisection (1906–1912), but the public, buoyed by such spectacular
medical advances as those described in Chapter 2, were less keen
to condemn all experimentation. The influence of abolitionist societies declined and, after World War I, groups with more moderate
goals rose to prominence. In 1926, the University of London Animal
Welfare Society (later to become the Universities Federation for
Animal Welfare (UFAW)) was formed by Major Charles W. Hume
(1886–1981). In 1962, Hume wrote that UFAW had been formed
in part

to compensate the harm done to the cause of animal welfare by animal-lovers of the unbalanced kind, and to form an intelligently humane body of public opinion. (Hume 1962, p. 202)

Notable among the achievements of this society was the publication in 1947 of the *UFAW Handbook on the Care and Management of Laboratory [and Other Research] Animals* (Eighth edition: Hubrecht and Kirkwood 2010). Of equal importance was the commissioning of William Russell and Rex Burch to write *The Principles of Humane Experimental Technique* (1959), a guide which pioneered the notion of the 'three Rs', namely: to seek *replacements* for animal experiments whenever possible; a *reduction* in the number of animals used in each procedure; and the *refinement* of experiments to eliminate wasteful or unnecessary procedures. (The 'three Rs' are considered in detail in Chapter 7.)

### BEYOND BRITAIN: OPPOSITION IN THE USA INTO THE TWENTIETH CENTURY

Medical research flourished throughout the western world in the twentieth century and perhaps nowhere more so than in the USA. Several factors perhaps contributed to the USA's successful medical research efforts. First, there were greater opportunities to obtain research funding, notably from philanthropic organisations. Leading from this, it can be argued that American scientists were paid more and had higher professional status (and concomitant skills and training) compared with their European colleagues. Second, the USA had, for the most part, a rapid and sustained economic growth in the twentieth century, while Europeans were impeded by the social and economic effects of two world wars fought on their soil. Finally (and the subject of discussion here), perhaps it was the lack of concerted opposition to animal experimentation which delayed federal animal protection legislation until the 1960s and left scientists free to perform certain experiments that could not be conducted elsewhere.

A key reason for this delay in the enabling of legislation may well have stemmed from the amount of animal-based research that had been conducted in the USA. Far fewer animal experiments had been performed before the middle of the nineteenth century when compared to Britain, and American public interest in vivisection and its opposition was scant.

Despite this, welfarists such as Henry Bergh (1811–1888), who had witnessed European animal experiments, tried to attract public support for the legislative control of vivisection in the USA. In 1866, Bergh founded the American Society for the Prevention of Cruelty to Animals (ASPCA), an organisation that was to argue unsuccessfully for the prohibition of vivisection in New York State in the 1870s. Following clashes in 1883 between welfarists and scientists in Boston and Philadelphia, some ASPCA members founded the abolitionist American Anti-Vivisection Society (AAVS) (Remfry 1987). Members and supporters of this organisation were successfully opposed by the National Academy of Sciences (NAS) and the American Medical Association (AMA), whose members argued for continued experimentation in an emerging era of major medical breakthroughs. Discoveries such as that of a diphtheria antitoxin in 1894 were embraced by an optimistic public excited by the promises of health and wealth that the new century was predicted to provide.

Arguably, the single event that was to determine the course of opposition to US medical research into the twentieth century took place in Washington, DC in 1896. Although the cries of anti-vivisectionist societies had gone largely unheard by the American public, concern that medical scientists may have been using animals in painful procedures did not escape the attention of some humanist welfare groups. Influential organisations such as the Women's Christian Temperance Union and the American Humane Association, together with the ASPCA, gained the support of a US senator in proposing legislation to Congress that aimed to restrict vivisection in the District of Columbia. Washington, DC was a major centre of medical research, and scientists saw in the proposed legislation restrictions that would impact the ways in which they could conduct research. Professional opposition to the proposed legislation was well organised through the AMA and NAS, providing medical testimony from American and British scientists promoting the benefits of animal-based research. In stark contrast to this professional approach, anti-vivisectionists only proffered old examples of vivisection derived from European practices. No attempt was made to illustrate their argument with contemporary American research that involved perceived cruelty, and the bill was defeated in the House of Representatives (Rowan and Rollin 1983; Rowan 1984; Lederer 1987).

This result set the scene for how animal experimentation would be viewed (and opposed) for the next 50 years. The public showed little interest in listening to animal welfare organisations, and when any such organisation looked like garnering any popular support, pro-vivisection groups such as the AMA's Committee for the Protection of Medical Research would counter with lobbying and propaganda (Benison 1970). In the face of the enormous strides taken by medical research and with a quiescent animal welfare lobby, American humanists and social reformers tended to turn their attentions elsewhere. At the 1914 American Humane Association conference a pro-research lobbyist was told that the association wished to 'leave vivisection alone' (Turner 1980, p. 118).

The use of animals in US biomedical research proliferated. Medical breakthroughs buoyed the biomedical industry and encouraged the use of animals in other scientific pursuits. Modern experimental psychology began a rise to prominence. With it came an enormous increase in the number of behavioural experiments that used animals as models of human conditions. Russian physiologist Ivan Pavlov (1849–1936) had been the first researcher to describe conditioned physiological responses to specific environmental stimuli. His famous experiments on the salivation responses of dogs contributed to a fundamental shift in emphasis for the causes of behaviour from internal mechanisms to environmental cues. At the same time as Pavlov, Englishman Edward Thorndike (1874–1949) had studied the reactions of hungry cats. Experimental subjects had been put into a 'puzzle-box' with food placed outside. A specified response (pushing a lever to unlock the door) allowed the cat to escape and feed. Thorndike reported that in early experiments, cats would obtain food through trial and error, but in later tests cats used learned behaviour (Poling et al. 1990).

In 1923, John Watson (1878–1958) introduced the works of Pavlov and Thorndike to the USA. He showed how such controlled experiments could be used to produce results that were both measurable and reproducible. Here was a rigorous scientific basis for psychology. Subsequently, experimental psychology extended the use of animals to studies that investigated memory, motivation, the interactions of mothers and their offspring, language and abnormal behaviour (Rowan 1984).

### The Animal Welfare Act

With increasing numbers of scientists using increasing numbers of animals (cats and dogs in particular), there came a point when demand was predicted to outstrip supply. Anticipating this, a pro-research group, the National Society for Medical Research, lobbied some US state politicians to guarantee a supply of animals through pounds and shelters. First Minnesota, then Wisconsin, New York, South Dakota, Oklahoma, Massachusetts, Connecticut, Utah, Ohio and Iowa passed pound-animal 'seizure' laws in the 1940s that legitimised the procurement of unwanted animals for experimentation (Rowan 1984). Cats and dogs that strayed or were placed in animal shelters could be taken by researchers for vivisection. The increased use of cats and dogs in experiments resulted in the 'uneasy truce' between humane societies and the research lobby being broken (Rowan 1984, p. 51). Cats and dogs are probably two animal species with which people most empathise, and animal welfare groups were able to convince the American Humane Association that such laws had to be repealed and that an appeal to public sensibilities would win the day. A new organisation, the Animal Welfare Institute (AWI), was set up by Christine Stevens in 1952 to fight for the rights of the unwanted pets. These were animals, it was argued, that ought to have been provided with sanctuary when they were no longer wanted, but now they were being sent to their deaths in research institutions. Initially, the AWI lacked the lobbying potential of the pro-experimentation groups, but by progressively appealing to public sentiment, its members were able to gather the kind of popular support that successful politicians are quick to recognise. AWI members toured research institutions and reported instances of inadequate care (Stevens 1990), further alerting an increasingly concerned public that the time for research animal welfare legislation was approaching.

Two pivotal events that occurred in the early 1960s were to result in the proclamation of such a law, the Federal *Laboratory Animal Welfare*

*Act* in 1966. Sixty years earlier in London a brown terrier 'done to death' had focussed public attention on the widespread use of dogs in British research (Ryder 2000). This time the concern of the US public was galvanised by the treatment of a Dalmatian called Pepper and an exposé by the populist *Life* magazine of the conditions in which starving dogs were kept by dog dealers in their pens (Mukerjee 1997). Pepper went missing and was thought by its owners to have been stolen and sold to a New York State dog dealer. Permission to visit the dealer's pens, first by the owners to confirm Pepper's identity and later by a congressman, was refused by the animal dealer and resulted in the politician (purportedly upset at the way he had been summarily dealt with by the dog dealer (Rowan 1984)) introducing legislation that was to regulate the trade in dogs. The Dalmatian was never positively identified as Pepper and was used for experimentation prior to euthanasia and incineration. Once again, however, in attaining martyrdom in the eyes of the public, an individual dog advanced the cause of laboratory animal welfare in a way that countless thousands that had died before it had been unable to do. By eliciting a widespread emotional response, Pepper's plight had focussed public and political attention on an aspect of animal experimentation that clearly warranted regulation.

A second event followed on from the Dalmatian's death. *Life* magazine (4 February 1966) published a photojournalistic article that exposed the shocking conditions under which dogs were kept by dealers prior to being sold for experiments. Public outrage ultimately resulted in federal legislation to license dealers and laboratories. In addition to licensing, the *Laboratory Animal Welfare Act* (1966) also required regular inspections of research facilities by the US Department of Agriculture (USDA) and accorded protection to cats, dogs, primates and rodents (in some circumstances). The Act was amended in 1970 (as the *Animal Welfare Act*) to include any category of warm-blooded animals except livestock. However, in 1971 the USDA excluded laboratory mice, rats and birds from the Act[1]. The Act was further amended in

---

[1] Despite long-term attempts by welfare organisations since 1971, rats and mice bred for research, amphibians and reptiles, all of which are given legislative protection in Britain, Europe, Canada, Australia and New Zealand, remain outside the US *Animal Welfare Act* (see Chapter 6).

1976 to require the use of post-operative analgesia. Further amendments in the 1980s and early 1990s established institutional animal care and use committees (IACUCs), required appropriate veterinary care, imposed exercise requirements for dogs, stated that experiments must minimise pain and distress, and instigated guidelines for the psychological well-being of primates. Inspectors from USDA now ensure that such issues are addressed and IACUC members now recognise these issues as significant IACUC-stated responsibilities.

As with the impetus for the enacting of the *Laboratory Animal Welfare Act* (1966), intense public attention, this time focussed upon the welfare of monkeys used in research, was to be the principal cause of amendments made in 1985. The 1960s and 1970s had been pivotal decades for the advancement of animal welfare in the United States and elsewhere. One reason for this involved increasing public support for civil and environmental movements in general. Activists were fast learning that in order to gather popular support for a cause, the interest of the media was essential. In 1981, television channels broadcast pictures of the confiscation by police officers of 17 monkeys from a Maryland research facility. These animals (16 crab-eating macaques and 1 rhesus macaque) became known as the Silver Spring monkeys. They had been used in research relevant to the rehabilitation of human stroke victims, research that involved the deadening of all nerves in the macaques' forearms (deafferentation). The research was designed to see how the monkeys altered their behaviour in response to the deafferentation. The monkeys treated their forearms as being foreign to them and, at the time the police confiscated them, individual animals had chewed off their fingers. Additionally, it was apparent that the animals had been mistreated: some had infected wounds, and the television crews were shown the filthy conditions in which the animals had been housed (Orlans 1993). Cruelty charges were brought against the administrative director of the research facility, and the National Institutes of Health ceased all relevant funding. The level of exposure this event received through the media resulted in enormous public sympathy for the cause of laboratory animal welfare.

Increasingly, it was learned by welfare activists that turning acts of civil disobedience into theatre was much more likely to receive television

coverage than passive protest or petition writing. This had direct consequences for the ways in which protests against animal experimentation
were to evolve (Goodman and Sanders 2011). In joining a moderate
organisation, concerned citizens only had recourse to moderate campaigns in order to initiate reform. In contrast, street demonstrations
and sit-ins were seen as much more likely to accelerate the process of
change. An extremist fringe believed they needed to go even further,
and civil disobedience gave way to criminal trespass in research institutions and, in some circumstances, the theft of laboratory animals.
One such act in 1984 resulted in the exposure of gross welfare abuses at
the University of Pennsylvania, where baboons were being used in
head-injury research (Orlans 1993). Subsequent media exposure of
stolen videotapes showing the details of particular procedures and
recording a total lack of regard for the welfare of individual baboons
resulted in massive popular support for a strengthening of the *Animal
Welfare Act* in 1985.

However, despite the 'ends-justify-the-means' approach of some activists, law-breaking of this kind was never to be viewed favourably by the
majority of the public, and illegal protests now are rarely, if ever, covered
by electronic media. A survey of animal rights demonstrators found that
criminal acts (including harassment of researchers and the liberation of
laboratory animals) were rated as the least effective methods of advancing
animal welfare. More effective methods were ranked as school education,
company boycotts, legal protection, setting personal examples, marches
and demonstrations (Galvin and Herzog 1998).

The 1970s and 1980s also saw increased interest in the welfare of
animals among moral philosophers. Perhaps the most influential work
to be published at that time, or since, was Australian philosopher Peter
Singer's *Animal Liberation* (1975). This book provided a rallying cry for
many opponents of animal experimentation by giving intellectual cre-
dence to what often had been criticised as sentimentality. Singer, reviv-
ing Bentham's utilitarianism, argued for the liberation of animals based
on *equality of consideration* and their capacity to suffer:

> [T]he fundamental common interest between humans and other
> animals remains the interest in not experiencing pain and suffering.

The only acceptable limit to our moral concern is the point at which there is no awareness of pain or pleasure, and no preferences of any kind. That is why the principle of equal consideration of interests has implications for what we may do to rats, but not for what we may do to lettuces. Rats can feel pain, and pleasure. Lettuces can't. (cited in Australian Government Senate Select Committee on Animal Welfare, 1989 p. 25)

Singer maintained that since laboratory animals were capable of feeling pain, their interests must be considered morally. His principle of equality of consideration insists that all sentient animals be given the same level of consideration in any moral calculation. If the level of suffering in an experiment involving sentient animals is not out-weighed by any increase in the quality of human life, it is morally indefensible to allow such an experiment to continue. However, an experiment may promise outstanding benefits that clearly outweigh the suffering of the experimental subjects. In such a case, a moral argument could be made for the experiment to proceed. Singer (1975) challenged scientists to argue that there was any difference between the moral status of human and non-human beings. If such a difference in moral status existed, how was it to be defined? If a difference could not be argued, how could scientists perform experiments on animals that they would not be prepared to conduct using humans?

Although the majority of animal researchers did not subscribe to Singer's arguments, *Animal Liberation* was pivotal in rekindling debate (which had lain dormant for much of the twentieth century) over the relative worth (costs versus benefits) of animal experimentation.

*Animal Liberation*, together with Richard Ryder's *Victims of Science* (1975) and, later, Bernard Rollin's *Animal Rights and Human Morality* (1981) were crucial publications in the resurgence of popular interest in the controversy that is animal welfare. These books were to focus public attention on clear instances where researchers were misusing animals in their care. The implication was that if research, such as that illus-trated by Singer (1975), Ryder (1975) and Rollin (1981), was being conducted in certain institutions, was it not reasonable to assume that similar things were going on elsewhere?

Popular novelists, too, incorporated research animal welfare into works of fiction to draw the attention of a broader readership to some of the poor experiments that had been conducted since the Second World War (see, for example, Richard Adams' *The Plague Dogs*, 1977). Scientists could no longer defend all experiments in the somewhat paternalistic ways of some of their predecessors. They were challenged to defend their practices in a philosophical arena and to demonstrate a morally relevant distinction between humans and other animals that could justify the use of one but not the other in laboratory experiments. In Chapter 4, Singer's and other major philosophical arguments that have contributed to these changes are presented in more detail. Chapters 5, 6 and 7 then illustrate the way in which modern science has responded to such challenges.

# 4   The moral status of animals

It is just not adequate for scientists to argue that there is a quantum difference between the moral status of humans and [other] animals if they are unable to give reasons for such a belief and defend their reasons in the arena of modern philosophical debate.

*Andrew N. Rowan (1984, p. 260)*

## ON THE MORAL STATUS OF ANIMALS

### Shaping the moral line

It is doubtful that any issue in science has generated as much emotion as animal experimentation did. In the previous chapter, readers were introduced to some of the historical reasons for the rise in opposition to vivisection. There had been three major components to criticism. First, how applicable to the human condition was scientific knowledge gained from experiments on non-humans? Early experiments, particularly prior to the discovery of anaesthetics, were crude and the results obtained were questionable. However, the use of increasingly sophisticated physiological techniques had led to a growing confidence in the reliability of experimental procedures. When this was coupled with a rigorous adherence to an evolving scientific method, the strength of this objection was reduced. Today, the dimensions and success of the biomedical industry attest to the acceptance and relevance of results gained from many species used as models of human conditions.

The second argument against vivisection had been based on the notion that, despite a prevailing Cartesian view among some experimenters that animals were incapable of feeling pain, cruel experiments were considered an affront to civilised (and predominantly) English sensibilities. The discovery of the anaesthetic properties of ether in the 1840s reduced support for this objection.

The third criticism of vivisection, endorsed by advocates of utilitarianism, that many animals were capable of suffering and therefore warranted *moral consideration*, was powerful. However, nineteenth-century anti-vivisectionists and twentieth-century animal welfarists were often viewed (and dismissed) as emotional animal lovers, unable to articulate their beliefs clearly in the face of authoritative science and medicine. It was not until the publication of central works by moral philosophers in the 1970s and 1980s that this situation was turned on its head. Philosophers such as Peter Singer (1975) challenged those who argued that there were fundamental differences in the moral status of human and non-human beings (and that these differences entitled them to exploit non-humans for the benefit of humanity) to show where the moral line between humans and other animals began and ended. In *Animal Liberation,* Singer (1975) highlighted incidences where animals were being exploited in industries as diverse as farm animal production, product testing and animal experimentation. He argued that, in the research arena, for example, the onus was on scientists to justify their experiments using, among other things, considered philosophical debate.

How does one measure the merits of a particular moral argument? Most scientists would admit to occupying a philosophical middle-ground somewhere between the protagonist who lobbies for the abolition of all research involving animals and the supporter of a research arena free from any form of regulation. More intensive questioning, however, may reveal a reluctance to elaborate on a chosen moral stance. The moral implications for anyone involved in animal research are complex, and most scientists (indeed, most people) are unsure of the solidity of their position in such a philosophical discussion. This has been the cause of some concern. Rather than adopt a moral viewpoint regarding their own work, some experimenters may choose to assume a low profile while waiting for public anxieties to be assuaged by colleagues (Cressey 2011). It has been suggested that some scientists, perhaps, fear a too-critical self-inquiry because it might reveal a weakness in their particular philosophical point of view (Britt 1984).

Of equal concern is the attitude of some scientists that, as long as they remain within regulatory boundaries, their research is their own responsibility and there is no need to be accountable publicly. For example, in a pamphlet published by the British Physiological Society's Education Sub-Committee (1983), physiological experiments involving animals were defended to young scientists. It was argued that physiologists should be guided by their consciences as to what was acceptable experimental technique, but that the goal of good science ought to be uppermost in their minds: 'animal experimentation poses ethical problems, because we are ourselves animals and we have, or possibly we imagine we have, empathy with other animals'. Arguments relating to a reduction in the numbers of animals used in experiments were dismissed: 'On moral pressures to use less [sic] animals, you and your colleagues in the scientific community are the only judges of the numbers needed. It is your reputation; you must stand firm' (cited in Langley 1989, p. 208).

Both the 'head-in-the-sand' stance and the 'rule-book scientist' point of view are, fortunately, becoming the exception rather than the rule as modern scientists move forward to grapple with the intricacies of con-temporary ethical debate.

The shaping of the moral line between humans and non-humans continues. Individual attitudes towards animals are diverse and shifting, and societal interchanges between humans and non-humans are complex. Today, every student and researcher involved in animal experimentation should consider a number of ethical questions. One such question will suffice to illustrate how difficult each is to answer. Many animals are used in experiments because they are so like us – this makes them good models of human conditions in biomedicine. But if these animals are so like us, why do we treat them so differently? To do so, Peter Singer (1978; 1990, pp. 27–91) argued, is to disregard their *interests*, while for Tom Regan (1981; 1982, pp. 363–394), it is in contravention of their *rights*.

This chapter examines Singer's and Regan's ethical arguments of animal 'interests' and animal 'rights' in detail. Their influence in modern debate is examined and the relative strengths and weaknesses of their arguments are highlighted. Additionally, further ethical view-points relevant to any discussion of the moral status of animals are outlined. First, humanism is described. Second, some have argued for an ethic not based exclusively on philosophical reason, but which also incorp-orates the emotionally derived concepts of empathy and compassion.

Such an ethic closely reflects the beliefs of Albert Schweitzer and the universality of his ideal of 'reverence for life' (Schweitzer 1936).

Despite genuine attempts by philosophers to achieve agreement about the width of the moral gulf between humans and other animals, no single ethical thesis has been universally accepted. This has important implications for debate about animal experimentation, where agreement would be invaluable. In the absence of such a consensus, some have proposed a form of practical moral stewardship by researchers for animals in their care. This also will be detailed.

As you will see, each ethical stance has its flaws, each has its critics. Nevertheless, each will serve to illustrate the breadth of the different opinions held in scientific and philosophical circles. Note, however, that while the points of view that follow are important in stimulating discussion, they must not be seen as the *only* ideas on the moral status of animals. Interested readers are referred to Stephen Clark's excellent coverage of further ideas in *The Moral Status of Animals* (1984) and *Animals and Their Moral Standing* (1997), and Lori Gruen's *Ethics and Animals: An Introduction* (2011) and *The Moral Status of Animals* (2014).

### Expanding the moral circle

What are ethics? What is morality? When we discuss ethics and morality, we refer to appropriate human conduct: what we ought to do, and why, in certain circumstances. *Ethic* is derived from the Greek *ethos*, meaning custom, people or system: *ethos* refers to the predominant community spirit. *Morality* is the distinction between right and wrong within that community spirit.

Historically in western communities, socially responsible human conduct has meant concern for others besides oneself and for the welfare of *human* society as a whole. Some philosophers and moral thinkers have argued for more expansive definitions. For example, early in the twentieth century, Albert Schweitzer examined prevailing anthropocentric ethical views (based in part on the thoughts of philosopher Immanuel Kant) and found them wanting. Schweitzer insisted that for the truly ethical person, *all* life (not just human life) was sacred and, therefore, worthy of moral consideration:

> [Ethics] must widen the circle from the narrowest limits of the family first to include the clan, then the tribe, then the nation and finally all mankind. But even when it has established the relationship between man and every other man it cannot stop. By reason of the quite universal idea ... of participation in a common nature, it is compelled to declare the unity of mankind with all created beings. (Schweitzer 1955, p. 261)

Others, including Aldo Leopold in *A Sand County Almanac* (1949), went further and argued for a comprehensive *environmental* ethic. Such an ethic (a 'land ethic') would incorporate not only life forms (human and non-human) but entire ecosystems, including the physical environment, the interactions between organisms, and between organisms and their non-living environment.

> The land ethic simply enlarges the boundaries of the [ethical] community to include soils, waters, plants and animals, or collectively, the land. (Leopold 1949, p. 219)

Enlarging the ethical community beyond the human sphere requires a total reconsideration of which features are morally relevant. In *The Rights of Nature*, Roderick Nash (1990, p. 4) recognised as 'one of the most extraordinary developments in recent intellectual history' the development of the relationship between humans and nature into an ethical one. He described, as Schweitzer had previously, how modern western ethics evolved from a pre-ethical past, where first the sphere of consideration was restricted only to the self. This had then expanded progressively to include kin, tribe and neighbours. Western ethical ideals over recent centuries have also urged a moral consideration of one's nation, one's race and finally all humanity. Nash predicted that the logical extension of ethical concern would next include all animals, then plants, all life, ecosystems, the planet and, finally, the universe.

It is one thing to make such a prediction, another to argue that it is defensible, desirable or justifiable. What we can see, though, is that before you and I can make a decision about an appropriate ethic of animal experimentation, we are confronted by differences of opinions about what sorts of ethics we could adopt as individuals. Kant was anthropocentric, i.e. human beings have a special value; Schweitzer argued that all life had moral relevance; for Leopold it was all life and ecosystems; and for Nash, perhaps, the entire universe. Whether we believe that appropriate human conduct involves only humans, or humans *and* certain mammals, or all animals *and* plants but not rocks, is something on which consensus is yet to be reached.

### MORAL ARGUMENTS BASED ON REASON

The redefining of a society's ethics and morals has generally coincided with historical turning points, such as emancipation from slavery. The twentieth century witnessed a continuation of this trend. The 1960s and 1970s were crucial decades for those committed to the ideal of freedom from discrimination for women and non-white races. A quantum extension of ethics was proposed when Peter Singer asserted in *Animal Liberation* (1975) that moral consideration must transcend the species boundary to include all sentient animals. Since then, contributions by philosophers to discussion of the moral status of animals and the consequences for their use for scientific purposes have been far-reaching. Reasoned intellectual debate has increasingly replaced the violent and illegal demonstrations thought necessary by some anti-vivisectionists, and has led to a reduction in insularity on the part of many researchers. Few scientists would now regard the criticisms of moderate welfarists as merely the rantings of ill-informed sentimentalists.

In order to clarify the moral issues which have been proposed as relevant to a discussion of animal experimentation, it is helpful to consider first a number of rationally based ethical stances.

### Humanist views

Today, few thinkers are willing to advocate the Cartesian view of humanism, that is, that all non-human animals are insentient and, therefore, incapable of feeling pain. However some, such as British psychologist Nicholas Humphrey, have offered their opinion that non-human animals are without self-consciousness:

> Descartes was as nearly right as makes no matter. If we walk down
> an English county lane, we walk by ourselves. Trees, birds, bees, the

rabbit darting down its hole, the cow heavy with milk waiting at the farmer's gate are all as without insight into their condition as the dummies on show at Madame Tussaud's. (cited in Rodd 1990, p. 42)

... and possibly without any form of consciousness:

> indeed we cannot be sure that animals consciously feel anything at all. Appearances notwithstanding, it is logically possible that animals are (as Descartes believed) merely unconscious automata. (Humphrey 1983, p. 42)

Such views are not widely held. Important studies of self-recognition using chimpanzees and mirrors have shown that some animals (other than humans) are capable of recognising themselves. Gordon Gallup (cited in Denton 1993, pp. 55–65) anaesthetised captive chimpanzees and, while they were unconscious, painted red markers above one eyebrow and the top of their opposite ear. The dye was odourless and positioned so that the chimps could not see that they had been marked. When each chimp regained consciousness, a mirror was introduced into its cage (one chimp, one mirror per cage; every individual had been exposed to mirrors prior to the experiment) and a careful score of the number of times each chimp touched the dye marker was kept. Gallup found that the number of times the area around the mark was touched rose 25-fold when compared with random touching prior to the introduction of the mirror. If a chimpanzee, on seeing its reflection, interpreted that reflection as another individual rather than itself, would not the chimp touch the mirror rather than its own head? As Derek Denton (1993, p. 60) concluded,

> you cannot examine otherwise-invisible portions of your body with the aid of a reflection unless you know who you are – that is, the animal is aware of itself.

If one is to argue that humans differ from non-humans because of our level of consciousness or self-consciousness, we must see that the difference is one only of degree, not of kind. If some primates other than ourselves are capable of some form of consciousness, what of others? If we are arguing over degrees of consciousness, has not the demarcation between humans and non-humans become just a little fuzzy?

A humanist might suggest other criteria which make humans worthy of ethical consideration, such as our advanced communication skills, or our (sometime) propensity to altruism, but critics will always counter all such reasons with examples from the animal kingdom. Carl Sagan and Ann Druyan (1992) are particularly adept at this.

Immanuel Kant (1724–1804) believed that appropriate human conduct (morality) did not extend beyond the human sphere because only humans were an end in themselves. All other animals were seen as a means to an end. He argued that overt cruelty to animals was to be avoided, not because humans had any form of duty to them, but rather because humans had indirect duties to humanity. Cruelty could never be defended, because 'he who is cruel to animals becomes hard also in his dealings with men' (cited in Infield 1963, p. 239).

This way of thinking perhaps had an earlier precedent in William Shakespeare's *Cymbeline*[1] (Act I, Scene V):

| Queen (addresses Cornelius): | I will try the forces of these thy [poisons] on such creatures as we count not worth the hanging, but none human... |
| --- | --- |
| Cornelius: | Your highness, shall from this practice but make hard your heart? |

Traditional Kantian humanism acknowledges that sentient animals are capable of suffering, but argues that all non-human animals lack the critical quality of moral autonomy or personhood which makes humans so unique. Without moral autonomy there can be no understanding of duty, so other animals, while worthy of our moral concern, cannot be afforded any moral status in their own right.

The problem with applying Kantian humanist theory to the practical day-to-day conduct of animal experiments does not involve the breadth of the moral divide between humans and non-humans. Rather, it is its failure to make a theoretical distinction between animal species *beyond* the human sphere. Consequently, this strictly humanist viewpoint can morally justify the use of a chimpanzee in an experiment where a laboratory rat would suffice, because neither species has moral autonomy.

[1] http://shakespeare.mit.edu/cymbeline/cymbeline.1.5.html

In all countries which have laboratory animal laws, however, the legislation and day-to-day regulation of animal experiments does not reflect this: both make hierarchical distinctions between non-human species (see further discussion in this chapter and Chapter 6).

### Singer and animal 'interests'

Around the same time as Kant, Jeremy Bentham ((1789) 1970, p. 283) alluded to an ethical expansion beyond the human domain when he asked of other animals: 'The question is not Can they *reason?* nor Can they *talk?*, but Can they *suffer?*' Peter Singer (1975) revived Bentham's utilitarian claim that equal consideration must be given to all beings that were capable of suffering, *based upon that capacity to suffer*. He adopted an ethical stance which has proved to be pivotal. He argued that moral judgements must be made based on equal interests and, in the same way as we should never be influenced by race or sex, we should never be influenced by species:

> If a being suffers, there can be no moral justification for refusing to take that suffering into consideration. No matter what the nature of the being, the principle of equality requires that its suffering be counted equally with the like suffering – in so far as rough comparisons can be made – of any other being. (Singer 2011, p. 50)

In other words, before taking any action which may involve distress, a utilitarian must perform a moral calculation. If an action (say, an animal experiment) leads to a net increase in the amount of 'good' for sentient (especially human) life, then that action is justified. If, however, a particular action causes more 'evil' for more sentient creatures than it produces 'good' for others, then that action is not justified.

Singer (1990) does not argue that all sentient species are of equal worth. Rather, as a *preference utilitarian*, he supports the idea that human beings, because of a combination of capacities which include self-awareness, acute intelligence, complex language and the ability to plan for the future, are entitled to specific preference for continued existence. Nevertheless, it is not possible to argue that smarter (or stronger) is better and therefore the use of less intelligent (or weaker) animals is justified. To adopt such a 'might makes right' attitude essentially invalidates all morality (Rowan and Rollin 1983). Nor does Singer (1990, p. 85) argue that his moral calculation will necessarily lead to the prohibition of all animal experimentation, because

> in extreme circumstances, absolutist answers always break down ... if a single experiment could cure a disease like leukemia, that experiment would be justifiable.

But Singer (1990, p. 85) does assert that

> in actual life the benefits are always more remote and more often than not they are non-existent ... an experiment cannot be justifiable unless the experiment is so important that the use of a brain-damaged human would also be justifiable.

Here, Singer is not advocating the use of people with severe intellectual disabilities in experiments (although this accusation was levelled at him: Singer 1993, pp. 337–359). His point is that it is morally indefensible to countenance experimentation using animals, rather than experimentation using humans with similar abilities to comprehend their situation, if the decision to use non-human animals is based on the subject of species difference. Singer (2011) argues that such a view is *speciesism* and is as unjustifiable in a moral community as racism or sexism.

### Regan and animal 'rights'

A third moral view, supported most strongly by Tom Regan (1981, 1982, 1983, 1985, 1990), involves animal *rights* (Gaughen 2005). Regan has proposed that the 'inherent value' of an individual (of any species) must be measured by its experience of the importance of its own life to itself. 'Inherent value' is the value of conscious individuals regardless of their usefulness to others, and independent of their 'goodness'. Equal rights for such individuals protect their 'inherent value' and give it (and them) moral status.

Regan has argued that any dealings which humans have with non-humans involve some exploitation of their rights. When it comes to animal experimentation, his views are unequivocal:

> [T]he rights view is categorically abolitionist ... This is just as true when [animals] are used in trivial, duplicative, unnecessary or unwise research as it is when they are used in studies that hold

out real promise of human benefits ... The best we can do when it comes to using animals in science is – not to use them. (Regan 1985, p. 24)

### Animal interests and animal rights: strengths

Of the moral views summarised above, the latter two have had the most impact on the way in which animal experiments are now conducted. In 1978, Singer predicted that the earlier publication of works by himself (Singer 1975), Regan and Singer (1976) and Richard Ryder (1975) would result in the elevation of debate beyond the unproductive arena of name-calling and ill-founded accusation, to the productive realm of reasoned philosophical debate (Singer 1978). The ideas put forward by Singer and Regan have provided a sensible departure point for debate over the moral issues essential in any rational discussion of animal experimentation. It has not been productive to counter logical philosophical arguments with rhetoric or emotional responses. The evolution of such arguments has led to meaningful dialogue between those who conduct experiments using animals and those who are concerned with animal welfare. Since Singer (1978) made his prediction, professional and popular support has indeed brought about a fundamental shift in the way in which non-human beings are perceived and has resulted in immeasurable improvements in the welfare of both laboratory and free-living animals used in research.

An example of this support for the expansion of ethics beyond the human sphere was reported by Nicholas Wade (1978) in the *Science* journal. An application was lodged by a pharmaceutical company with the US Fisheries and Wildlife Service to import chimpanzees (an endangered species) into the USA from Sierra Leone in the mid-1970s. It was intended that these chimpanzees would be used to test a potential vaccine against the virus which causes human hepatitis B. It was known that the capture of juvenile chimpanzees often involved the shooting of their mothers by uncaring trappers, but at that time about 1500 people were dying each year from hepatitis B in the USA. Wade (1978, p. 1030) concluded:

> The world has a growing population of [then] four billion people and a dwindling population of some 50,000 chimpanzees. Since the

vaccine seems unusually innocuous, and since the disease is only rarely fatal, it would perhaps be more just if the larger population could find some way of solving its problem that was not to the detriment of the smaller.

Many people, including members of an order of monks, volunteered to have trials conducted on them rather than on chimps. The application to use chimpanzees in this research was opposed by, among others, the International Primate Protection League and was rejected, principally because of an ethical stance that urged that threatened wildlife species should not be used in safety testing (Rolston 1988).

A rise in professional interest in what is termed 'compassionate conservation' reflects this growing concern for the welfare of free-living wildlife (Bekoff 2013). An individual wild animal's immediate welfare interests are being weighed against the potential of long-term conservation gains for populations or species (e.g. Hodgson and Koh 2016; Lindsjö, Fahlman and Törnqvist 2016; Waugh and Monamy 2016).

A good example of compassionate conservation involves the ban on hot iron branding of seals and sea lions on sub-Antarctic islands and elsewhere by the Australian and New Zealand governments (Monamy 2007). Conservation biologists had been hot iron branding seal and sea lion pups as a means of long-term identification for some years before it was brought to the attention of the wider community following widespread television exposure of the practice. Hot iron branding has long been used as a method of identification for cattle and horses, but the application of a hot iron to the protected hides of iconic wildlife species forced many people to confront the kind of dilemma which arises when arguments can be made for the moral 'rightness' of both sides of a debate. This was no simple calculation, such as when one weighs a moral 'right' against a moral 'wrong'. Rather, this controversy threatened the continuation of long-term conservation projects (wildlife research is popularly perceived as a moral 'good') because of the use of an identification technique often viewed as a 'necessary evil' when used on farms. Hot iron branding of baby sea lions caused a level of moral uneasiness which forced government bans and an evaluation of the relative importance of the kinds of wildlife studies which could only be conducted at the expense of *individual* animal welfare. Following the ban, welfare-neutral identification techniques such as unique whisker spot patterns in sea lions have been developed (Osterrieder *et al.* 2015).

### Animal interests and animal rights: weaknesses

The views of both Singer and Regan have not been immune to criticism, notably for polarising debate. Additionally, Singer's style of preference utilitarianism has been criticised for its lack of consistency. Moral calculations become tortuous and impractical when all factors are taken into consideration. Just how do you quantify an amount of pleasure or pain? James Battye (1994) considered the application of utilitarianism to the Roman Colosseum, where Christians were being used for sport. A 'do-gooder' complains to the Emperor that such practice is evil: 'Evil?' says the Emperor, 'That's easily fixed: we'll sell more tickets' (Battye 1994, p. 5.) The point Battye is emphasising is that an act considered 'evil' can be negated so long as you can increase the 'good' that it also brings about.

Tom Regan (1982, p. 46) also has argued that 'the animal industry is big business'. What he meant was that biomedicine employs hundreds of thousands of people who, in turn, have hundreds of thousands of dependants. A preference utilitarian (such as Singer) must take into consideration the interests of all such people if one is to advocate the reduction or closure of the industries which use research animals. Under Singer's terms, aren't such people's interests (in being employed and able, therefore, to support their families) of more importance than those of the research animals?

Regan's unshakeable beliefs in moral rights based on unquantifiable 'inherent value' have also been challenged on numerous grounds. Some claim, for example, that rights can be attributed only to individuals who can claim them, and that they can only apply in circumstances where that individual understands the notions of rights (i.e. only some humans: Smith and Boyd 1991). Regan has countered by pointing out that such a viewpoint would withhold rights from infants, the intellectually disabled and the senile. Do not all humans have the same rights?

> Animals, it is true, lack many of the abilities humans possess. They can't read, do higher mathematics, build a bookcase or make *baba*

*ghanoush*. Neither can many human beings, however, and yet we don't (and shouldn't) say that they (these humans) therefore have less inherent value, less of a right to be treated with respect, than do others. (Regan 1990, pp. 184–185; Regan's italics).

Others have attacked the absence of a clear distinction between 'moral' and 'legal' rights for individual animals of all species. Not all species have moral rights, and only one has legal rights (see Wise 2000, 2002 for a summary of this argument).

Further criticism deals with Regan's criterion for a claim to inherent value (and hence membership within a moral circle): 'Inherent value belongs equally to those who are the experiencing subjects-of-a-life' (Regan 1990, p. 186). To satisfy this criterion, an animal must be, among other things, conscious, have the capacities necessary to conceive the future, and to act deliberately. According to Regan, the only beings which satisfy this criterion are 'mentally normal *mammals* of a year or more [in age]' (Regan 1983, p. 78: my italics). J. Baird Callicott (1989, pp. 39–47) was especially critical of this feature of the 'animal rights' thesis. (Why not 'mammal rights?') In particular, Callicott (1989, pp. 40–41) criticised Regan's ecological naïveté. He referred to the following two passages from Regan's *The Case for Animal Rights* (1983) as evidence of the general inapplicability of the rights concept to biological conservation:

> Species are not individuals, and the rights view does not recognize the moral rights of species to anything, including survival. (Regan 1983, p. 359);

and:

> That an individual animal is among the last remaining members of a species confers no further right on that animal, and its rights not to be harmed must be weighed equitably with the rights of any others who have this right. If, in a prevention situation, we had to choose between saving the last two members of an endangered species or saving another individual who belonged to a species that was plentiful but whose death would be a greater prima facie harm to that individual than the harm that death would be to the two, then the rights view requires that we save that individual. (Regan 1983, p. 359)

Callicott (1989) argued that Regan had not considered that the vast majority of endangered species were in fact plants and insects and neither group could claim 'subjects-of-a-life' status according to Regan's criteria. Callicott suggested that if one had to choose between protecting the last two individuals of an endangered plant species from grazing by a starving rabbit (a plentiful species), then Regan would argue that the rights of an adult rabbit (a mammal) must override the absence of rights of the endangered plants.

Such a moral viewpoint advocating rights only for mammals is not a workable ethic for use in modern biology and has largely been set aside in contemporary debate.

Others are also critical of utilitarianism as it applies beyond the human sphere. For some, it simply does not go far enough – there is more to life, any life, than just pleasure and pain. Eminent Australian scientist and philosopher Charles Birch (1993, pp. 86–96) posed an interesting question: If all animals used for human purposes were to be constantly anaesthetised for all of their lives, thereby eliminating the pleasure/pain argument, would such a procedure be morally defensible? This is an excellent illustration of the differences which exist between animal *welfare* and animal *ethics*. Welfare issues for animals which, hypothetically, were to lead unconscious lives would be minimal, but the ethical issues associated with countenancing such an action are serious. Many people would hold intrinsic ethical objections to denying animals the opportunity to experience their own lives (Gott and Monamy 2004).

A rise in the number of procedures that involve the genetic alteration of laboratory animals has also highlighted another ethical issue that is not easily reconciled by the 'animal interests' and 'animal rights' theses of Singer and Regan. Research involving genetic alteration results in the directed breeding of many generations of animals (principally mice), of which the majority of offspring (>70%: Ormandy, Dale and Griffin 2011) do not have the desired genetic change. Animals without the desired phenotype and/or genotype may be deemed 'surplus' and are usually killed very early in their lives. This adds up to many millions of 'surplus' animals being killed each year worldwide (Taylor *et al.* 2008; UK Home Office 2016). Is it ethical to generate and then kill millions of 'surplus' animals in this way, even if their welfare interests (in a rapid and humane death) are met? Singer's 'interests' and Regan's 'rights' do not necessarily argue for consideration of the moral status of newborn laboratory mice.

ETHICS: ROOM FOR EMOTION?

**Empathy**

So why can't philosophers agree? Are all animals worthy of moral consideration? What about just sentient ones? But then where does sentience begin? How are we supposed to form a belief if the professionals cannot?

In an important contribution to ethical debate, Lori Gruen (1991) hinted that the apparent lack of agreement among philosophers perhaps was based on their use of reason *in the absence of emotion*. Gruen proposed that although any argument based solely on emotion was not able to be defended morally, it was also plausible that any ethical stance based exclusively on reason may be equally invalid. John Fisher (1987), too, has advocated that difficulties in arriving at agreement on the moral status of animals may have been exacerbated by not considering the concept of sympathy. He argued simply that any being worthy of sympathy must also be worthy of moral consideration:

> One of the most important reasons why sympathy is of interest to moral theory lies in the way that it determines the range of application of our moral intuitions. Our sympathetic response to animals makes them a part of our moral community; that is, our moral concerns and our ideas of right and wrong action extend to animals as well as to fellow humans. (Fisher 1987, p. 199)

This is especially relevant for animal researchers. If we agree that scientists, as moral stewards (see below), have obligations to their experimental subjects, but that no-one is absolutely sure where such responsibilities begin and end, how may we define appropriate behaviour or proper human conduct? In short, what must we do to derive an ethic of animal experimentation? Feeling sympathy with (or perhaps, empathy for) the subjects of our research is a concern born of emotionality, but scientific objectivity demands a rigorous *rational* approach to experimentation. This must create a tension between one's personal beliefs and one's professional behaviour. Might not such a tension be seen as beneficial when viewed within the framework of a universal ethic which has room for both rationality and emotionality? Such a framework is found in Albert Schweitzer's ethic of *der Ehrfurcht vor dem Leben,* or *reverence for life*.

### Reverence for life

Albert Schweitzer (1875–1965), Nobel Peace Laureate, medical practitioner, doctor of philosophy and theology, was committed to developing a universal ethic which could incorporate emotionality but which would be based on logic. Instead, in a flash of insight, he realised that the opposite would be the case: an ethic which advocated goodness towards all life, not just to humanity, would be derived, not from rational thought, but from emotion:

> Certain truths originate in feeling, others in the mind. Those truths that we derive from our emotions are of a moral kind – compassion, kindness, forgiveness. Reason, on the other hand, teaches us the truths that come from reflection ... The problem presented itself to me in these terms: must we really be condemned to live in this dualism of emotional and rational truths? ... does the mind, in its striving for a morality that can guide us in life, lag so far behind the morality that emotion reveals because it is not sufficiently profound to be able to conceive what the great teachers, in obedience to feeling, have made known to us?
>
> This led me to devote myself entirely to the search for a fundamental principle of morality ... I had to consider the question of what the fundamental idea of existence is. What is the mind's point of departure when it sets itself to the task of reflecting on humanity and on the world in which we live? This point of departure, I said to myself, is not any knowledge of the world that we have acquired. We do not have – and we will never have – true knowledge of the world; such knowledge will always remain a mystery to us.
>
> The point of departure naturally offered for meditation between ourselves and the world is the simple evidence that *we are life that*

*wishes to live and are animated by a will in the midst of other lives
animated by the same will.* Simply by considering the act of thinking,
our consciousness tells us this. True knowledge of the world consists in our being penetrated by a sense of the mystery of existence
and of life.

If we proceed on the basis of this knowledge, it is no longer
isolated reason that devotes itself to thought, but our whole being,
that *unity of emotion and reflection that constitutes the individual.*
(excerpt from radio interview, Radio Brazzaville (1955) cited in
Brabazon 1976, pp. 245–246: my italics)

Schweitzer's 'revelation' led to his writing of *Civilisation and Ethics*
(1955). It contained the fundamental principle which was, henceforth, to
govern all of his actions – reverence for life. This was an ethic which
affirmed for him the position of the human species in the universe.
This is further emphasised in *My Life and Thought* (1966):

> The most immediate fact of man's consciousness is the assertion:
> I am life which wills to live in the midst of life which wills to live . . .
> If man affirms his will-to-live, he acts naturally and honestly . . . [he]
> feels a compulsion to give to every will-to-live the same reverence for
> life that he gives to his own . . . He accepts as being good: to preserve
> life, to promote life, to raise to its highest value life which is capable
> of development. (Schweitzer 1966, pp. 130–131)

Reverence for life is a creed which makes no distinction between
'higher' or 'lower' life forms; no distinction between plants and animals;
no distinction between human beings and non-human beings. An
acceptance of such an ethic does not mean that causing the death of
another creature is wrong, it is the causing of pain or death *when it can be
avoided* that is wrong. Anyone guided by 'reverence for life' will only
cause the death or suffering of any animal in cases of *inescapable
necessity*, never from thoughtlessness. For Schweitzer, this had particular
relevance for the animal researcher:

> Those who experiment with operations or the use of drugs upon
> animals, or inoculate them with diseases, so as to be able to bring
> help to mankind with the results gained, must never quiet misgiv-
> ings they feel with the general reflection that their cruel proceedings

aim at a valuable result. They must first have considered in each individual case whether there is a real necessity to force upon any animal this sacrifice for the sake of mankind. And they must take the most anxious care to mitigate as much as possible the pain inflicted. (Schweitzer 1936, p. 252)

It is worth noting here that the use of the English word 'reverence' does not necessarily carry the full meaning of the German noun *Ehrfurcht*. James Brabazon (1976) doubted that 'reverence' instilled a full sense of mystical awe. He suggested that *Ehrfurcht* was ultimate respect, and should instil in us the sorts of feelings that we experience, for example, on top of mountains or in storms at sea. Put simply, a sense of the numinous.

Schweitzer's ethic is essentially theological, and has been criticised as being too simplistic for a world view, and impractical in any reasoned discussion of animal experimentation (Flemming 1984; Anon 1992). Peter Singer (1979) once pointed out that Schweitzer, as a physician, would have had little compunction in killing lower life forms, such as bacteria and parasites, in his treatment of patients. However, I would argue that Singer's criticism does not apply in any practical sense in the discussion of animal experimentation. Debate (and the focus of this book) is concentrated essentially on the welfare of those animals which are generally accepted as sentient beings (i.e. the animals with which we most empathise). This is reflected in the laws which govern experiments in western countries (see Chapter 6): they only apply to such clearly sentient animals. Researchers who experiment on creatures not considered sentient (i.e. all invertebrates except certain cephalopods) are not answerable to animal ethics committees or government inspectors. These laws mirror the fact that, for most people, concern for the welfare of animals in experiments is hierarchical (Mather 2011). Moral indignation and public outcry are invariably heightened when debate turns from, say, a discussion of the welfare of gut bacteria or insects to one of cats, dogs, sea lions or primates.

This is not to say that researchers using invertebrates need not necessarily operate under the same ethic. Anyone who has observed the behaviour of an octopus will understand that it is not only vertebrates that are sentient:

> [T]he octopus, a mollusc, is much closer genetically to a snail than a mouse is to me [but] appears to have a lot to communicate. If I approach an octopus, it looks at me, dilates its pupils, raises goose bumps on its skin, blushes and goes white and, if I persist, squirts ink at me. (Wall 1992, p. 1)

Concern for the welfare of the octopuses in scientific research resulted in an amendment to the UK *Animals (Scientific Procedures) Act* (1986) to include legal protection for *Octopus vulgaris* in 1993. Similar protection is offered in Australia (National Health and Medical Research Council 2013) and Canada to octopuses and squid (Wong 1995).

It is also interesting to note that in 1881 Charles Darwin ((1881) 1985) wrote an entire book on intelligence in earthworms, believing them to be able to make decisions in experimental mazes. Did Darwin, perhaps, recognise that the boundary between intelligent and non-intelligent animals may have less to do with the presence of a backbone than is generally believed? Our demarcation between vertebrates and invertebrates is a relatively recent taxonomic division. Intelligence was never a consideration when this division was made.

Elwood (2011) discussed whether insects were capable of experiencing pain. Earlier, Eisemann *et al.* (1984, p. 167) concluded that entomologists ought to inactivate insect nervous systems prior to trauma. In so doing, their subjects are not only easier to handle, but it instils in the researcher

> an appropriately respectful attitude towards living organisms whose physiology, though different, and perhaps simpler than our own, is as yet far from completely understood.

Singer (2011) argued that only *sentient* animals must be given an equality of consideration – a rational argument. Schweitzer urged that *all* life must be afforded the same respect: the need for every experiment must be carefully reasoned based on the ideal of reverence for life, not sentience – an argument that gives a place to emotion. Both points of view are entirely valid in the choosing of an ethic to govern animal experimentation. The Schweitzerian ideal, perhaps, has the potential to include animals excluded by Singer's sentience cut-off in the event that public pressure were to increase for the inclusion of more invertebrates covered by the legislative umbrellas currently governing animal experiments.

David Porter (1992, p. 101) courageously suggested that all scientists adopting the 'Schweitzerian' model may become 'anti-vivisectionists at heart.' The adoption of such an ethical stance would lead to the deliberate creation of tension between one's work and one's values. Porter (1992, p. 101) admitted that many researchers would find this an outrageous scenario, but emphasised that the 'onus is on them to explain why [scientists] would not want to share an ideal that seeks always to minimise or avoid the harm we inflict on sentient animals'.

### MORAL STEWARDSHIP

The four moral arguments described above, though helpful in the formation of an acceptable ethic of animal experimentation, tend to drift further and further away from the day-to-day reality of modern experimental procedures. Philosophers urge that the ability to make moral decisions ought to be an essential criterion in today's scientist. Few would disagree, and yet one is left with the notion that in the absence of an all-encompassing ethic of animal experimentation, there is little that is clear-cut and much that is various shades of grey. Another solution? Margaret Stone (1989, pp. 30–31), an academic lawyer who gave evidence before the Australian Government's Senate Select Committee on Animal Welfare (1989), was critical of the ability of any general moral principle to answer specific questions about what to do in individual cases of animal experimentation. For her, pragmatism was of far greater importance than finding a universally applicable ethic for use when considering research animals:

> [T]here are no simple answers to be found and there is no single guiding principle that will answer the questions that are raised about the problems of animal welfare and the use of animals in our society. There have been ... laudable attempts, which have had very many beneficial results, to provide such a principle but they have all failed. One reason why they have failed ... is that where ethical principles are concerned, there is no possibility of proving the validity of an ethical principle and that a single principle does not take account of what I would see as the competing interests of humans and animals ... So it seems to me that we have to move on very quickly from that ill-fated

search to find a single principle and get down to the nitty-gritty of trying to resolve problems that arise in particular instances.

A multidisciplinary working party convened by the British Institute of Medical Ethics (Smith and Boyd 1991) reviewed contemporary philosophical and moral debate about animal experimentation and arrived at the same conclusion. This committee consisted of veterinarians, scientists, moral philosophers and animal welfare group representatives. They agreed that if the current discrimination between humans and other animals as research subjects was justifiable, then a *relevant* difference between the moral status of humans and non-humans must be (a) alleged and (b) morally supported. Despite extensive and rigorous philosophical debate, they were unable to find agreement among philosophers on whether any difference between humans and non-humans *could* be supported morally:

> In the light of these conclusions, it is not surprising that the multidisciplinary Working Party responsible for this study is unable to offer arguments for or against the use of animals in biomedical research to which philosophers will not take exception. (Smith and Boyd 1991, p. 306)

In the absence of a keenly sought universal ethic of animal experimentation, sensible animal welfarists, both within science and without, have plotted a different course: many now recognise that animal researchers have a role as *moral stewards*. They do not object to animal experiments in situations where the research subjects are treated humanely and the experiments are justifiable because they contribute to the preservation or enhancement of human or non-human life. In this context, animal experimentation is viewed as a 'necessary evil' (Smith and Boyd 1991, p. 345), which is justifiable so long as those who conduct the experiments are in tune with their moral obligations – to society *and* to the animals in their care.

For supporters of moral stewardship, what has been established beyond doubt is that

> human beings bear the burden of ... respecting and protecting the interests and welfare of those creatures which are alive and do have

minimal levels of sentience ... Both the capacity for a full mental life and the ability to suffer place demands on the responsible moral [steward] that are sufficient in themselves to demand compliance and discharge. Animals deserve no less respect than that which we accord the most helpless and vulnerable members of our own species. (Caplan (1989), cited in Australian Government Senate Select Committee on Animal Welfare, 1989, p. 41)

## SUMMARY

We have examined several moral standpoints which involve our treatment of non-human beings in general and research animals in particular. The first, essentially Kantian ethic justifies our current use of animals based on a human uniqueness; the second, third and fourth points of view of Singer, Regan and Schweitzer, respectively, argue strongly for an expansion of our moral circle, but for different reasons. Many variations on this theme have been put forward in the past 40 years. Most of these ideas have merit of some kind, but none of them is sufficiently all-encompassing to make a decision about the moral value of all animals a simple one.

Irrespective of whether their particular moral stance holds in every case, it would be unfair to discount the contributions made by Peter Singer and others in elevating debate and drawing public attention to the conditions under which research involving animals is conducted. Most researchers using animals now recognise that they have to work within a moral framework determined by society as a whole, not exclusively by scientists (Monamy 2007).

The issues involved in the determination of the moral status of non-human animals are complex – yet they are at the heart of the animal experimentation debate. Each reader must attempt to form an opinion of his or her own about the extent to which we use research animals. To do so is not a simple task – it will involve rational discussion and personal feelings. Many of you would have serious misgivings if asked to experiment upon a cat or a dog in a practical class. Fewer have the same misgivings when dealing with other species, say, rats and mice. Yet, are not the rodents worthy of the same consideration?

Animal experimentation has been termed 'a necessary evil' (Smith and Boyd 1991, p. 345): an 'inescapable necessity' is, perhaps, less judgemental. It has numerous benefits for human and non-human health; it assists in the accumulation of ecological information necessary for species conservation in a world of dwindling natural habitat; and it provides many human societies with an array of commercial products, such as shampoos and cosmetics that consumers demand, safe for human use. At the same time, it causes pain and distress for millions of animals, whether purpose-bred, captured from the wild or collected as unwanted pets.

If animal experimentation is viewed as an 'inescapable necessity', questions can be asked immediately about how we can reduce the level of suffering inherent in some experiments. Are there alternatives to some procedures? Can we reduce the number of experiments of dubious value? Such questions are addressed in Chapters 5, 6 and 7.

# 5    Animal use

> Where there is no scientifically and morally acceptable alternative,
> some use of animals in biomedical research can be justified (albeit by
> different moral reasons for different people) as necessary to safeguard
> and improve the health, and to alleviate the suffering, of human beings
> and [other] animals; as well as to advance fundamental scientific
> knowledge, upon which such therapeutic and practical benefits might
> depend. Such a justification, however, should be considered very
> carefully indeed.
>
> *Smith and Boyd (1991, p. 329)*

## HOW ARE ANIMALS USED?

At the end of Chapter 2, I listed some of the numerous medical
advances that have been made through research involving animals.
It is not just the field of medicine in which such strides have been
taken, and it is worthwhile to consider more fully the extent to which
animals are used.

## FUNDAMENTAL AND APPLIED BIOLOGICAL RESEARCH

Fundamental, or pure, research aims to advance knowledge without
having specific aims, such as an improvement in human and non-
human health, in mind. Francis Bacon (1561–1626) eloquently described
such research as *experimenta lucifera*, or 'experiments which shed light'.
In contrast, *experimenta fructifera* described 'experiments which yield
fruit' (Paton 1993). Today's term for goal-directed experimentation is
'applied research'. In practice, pure research and applied research are
often inextricably linked. Fundamental investigations often result in
practical applications while applied efforts often lead into new areas of
fundamental research.

In biomedicine, 'illuminating' practices include experiments designed
to clarify physiological systems at the molecular, genetic and cellular

levels as well as at the level of organs or whole animals. Beyond biomedicine, in zoological studies, for example, fundamental research may include field-based studies of wild animal behaviour with a view to a greater understanding of biological processes or ecological interactions. Basic information of this kind may then be applied to determine an effective and humane way of controlling particular wildlife species that may have become pests (Littin 2010) or to conserve threatened species (Paul *et al.* 2015).

In applied biomedical research, animals are used in many ways. Sometimes a particular non-human species may be found that can act as an accurate model of a human disease. Research efforts then may be expanded to include experimentation with this species to complement ongoing research involving humans. One such example is Pompe's Disease (generalised glycogenosis, type II), an inherited, lethal, lysosomal storage disease afflicting some human infants in their first year of life (van der Ploeg and Reuser 2008). In Western Australia, a herd of Shorthorn cattle was found to produce calves with generalised glycogenosis, type II. Affected calves showed syndromes similar to those observed in clinically ill human sufferers (Di Marco, Howell and Dorling 1984). These animals provided an opportunity to determine ante-natal and post-natal changes associated with the disease in humans and were used to develop enzyme replacement techniques to assist in therapy and prevention (Howell, Dorling and Cook 1983).

In other applied studies, organs may be required from experimental animals, or animals might be needed to test the efficiency and safety of vaccines. For example, in the first half of the twentieth century, monkeys were integral to the research that resulted in the development of vaccines against poliomyelitis. Polio is an infectious viral disease that causes paralysis and muscle wastage in children. In 1909, scientists had discovered that the polio virus was transferable to some species of monkeys (Flexner and Lewis 1909). This meant that many investigations which, for contemporary ethical reasons, could not be conducted using human subjects could now proceed with monkeys. Forty years later, research had advanced to the stage where researchers successfully cultured the virus on human tissue (Enders, Weller and Robbins 1949). This led to a vaccine being released in 1955. Its effect in reducing the number of polio cases was spectacular. During a polio epidemic in 1952, 58 000 cases were reported in the USA. In 1984, only four cases were recorded throughout the USA (US Congress, Office of Technology Assessment 1986). In 1988, the World Health Organization launched the Global Polio Eradication Initiative. Since then there has been a >99 per cent reduction in infection rates worldwide (Kew 2012).

In order to mass-produce the vaccine, monkey kidney tissue was needed to produce large quantities of the virus. This meant that many monkeys were sacrificed for their kidneys. Other live monkeys were necessary to test the safety of the vaccine. Today, monkeys are no longer used in the propagation of viruses for vaccine production, although they are still used in safety testing (Rubin 2011).

### GENETIC ALTERATION

An area of scientific research involving animals which has undergone extraordinary growth in the past 25 years has been transgenesis and cloning. Transgenesis and cloning are forms of genetic modification where an organism's genetic code is altered to induce mutation so that gene function may be investigated. Genetic alteration can occur naturally at any time (e.g. immuno-compromised mice), but targeted mutagenesis and transgenesis allow researchers to study the deliberate under-expression or over-expression of specific genes. In transgenesis, genetic material from one species (e.g. a human protein) may be inserted into another (e.g. a cow). Targeted mutagenesis results in specific genes being made functional ('knocked-in') or non-functional (knocked-out'). Cloning is where a nucleus from a body tissue cell replaces the nucleus of an enucleated egg cell. The modified cell is then implanted into the uterus of a surrogate mother and pregnancy continues, resulting in the birth of a near copy of the original donor animal. Animal models reliant upon such forms of genetic alteration have been used to shed light on the pathology of many human diseases, particularly arthritis, cancer, diabetes and heart disease.

In 1992, transgenic research involved less than 1 per cent of research animals worldwide, but in 2001, 20 per cent of research protocols involving animals were in transgenic research (Mitchell 2001). By 2005, the UK Home Office reported that nearly one million regulated procedures in Britain involved the use of genetically altered animals, representing a third of all scientific procedures involving animals (UK Home Office 2007). By 2015, the total number of completed procedures exceeded four million, with half involving genetically altered animals (UK Home Office 2016).

Rapid advances in genome editing technologies (particularly CRISPR/Cas9: Riordan *et al.* 2015) hold the promise of more precisely targeted genetic alterations (Singh, Schimenti and Bolcun-Filas 2015) that could result in fewer animals being needed. However, the ease and relative low cost of new gene drive technologies could also result in more researchers using genetic alteration (Nuffield Council on Bioethics 2016). There could also be a trend towards further increases in research animal numbers because of the use of species other than mice and zebrafish (Seruggia and Montoliu 2014). Recent applications of genome editing in combination with pluripotent stem cells to grow organs from one species (humans) in another species (pigs) offers an example of this (Feng *et al.* 2015).

For the first time since the mid-1970s, the total number of animals used for experimentation has begun to increase. Overwhelmingly, the animal most used, accounting for 98 per cent of all procedures, is the laboratory mouse. Enormous breeding programmes are required to generate heterozygous strains of mice with genetic modifications, and entirely new ethical concerns relating to husbandry and welfare have become apparent (Bruce and Bruce 2003; Buehr, Hjorth and Hansen 2003; Wells *et al.* 2006; Ormandy, Dale and Griffin 2011; Behrens 2014).

Many of the animals involved in genetic alteration procedures are not used for experimentation (UK Home Office 2016). Rather, they are the progeny of the few animals being used to continue a genetically modified strain. Such individuals may have no conspicuous phenotypic changes and are deemed to be 'surplus'. Nevertheless, these animals also have welfare needs which must be addressed.

Individuals which are born with a successful genetic modification will often show phenotypic changes resulting from the altered genotype. Change to an animal's phenotype may involve altered physiology and anatomy. Such changes can have unintended (or intended) welfare consequences and have led to widespread concern about the overall well-being of such research animals (Bilbo and Nelson 2001; Bailey, Rustay and Crawley 2006; Brown and Murray 2006; Behrens 2014). This is also of particular relevance to genetically altered farm animals where lifetime monitoring may be necessary to detect gene expression at any stage of an animal's life (Animal Welfare Committee 2007).

## BEHAVIOURAL RESEARCH

Behavioural researchers may use animals in order to understand more completely human psychological phenomena. Animals have been used in diverse research areas including depression, drug addiction, aggressive behaviour, communication, learning and problem solving, normal and abnormal social behaviour, reproduction and parental care. Such research varies widely in its effects on the animals themselves. Experiments may be as innocuous as the non-intrusive study of behaviour in wild animals or, for instance, observing the responses of free-living vervet monkeys to the playback of recorded intraspecific alarm calls (Seyfarth, Cheney and Marler 1980). Conversely, some animals have been subjected to repeated exposure to painful stimuli, such as inescapable electric shock, or have been harmed psychologically in experiments examining the effects of maternal deprivation (Rowan 1984; Stephens 1986).

## EDUCATION AND TRAINING

Many students are exposed to animals and animal dissection at some stage during their schooling. Primary education may offer opportunities for children to interact with small animals (usually insects, mammals and birds) and so develop a positive attitude towards them. Students are encouraged to care for classroom pets and to observe general behaviour patterns. During secondary schooling, students may be exposed to animal dissection using amphibians or rodents. Senior high school students may even conduct non-invasive behavioural experiments of their own using, for example, finches or mice. An education that includes exposure to the humane care of animals may have positive effects later, when many university life science students are exposed to animal experimentation. As undergraduates, they may find themselves actively experimenting with animals of varying sentience, to gain knowledge and to acquire specialised skills. Involvement in experimentation will vary depending on the course in which a student is enrolled. Students of the medical and allied health professions (e.g. physiotherapy, dentistry) as well as veterinary and agricultural science students, usually receive 'vocational' training. As such, experiments using animals will be restricted to those that illustrate a particular concept or identify a particular physiological system. Students of more 'research orientated' professions (e.g. genetics, physiology, zoology, pharmacology, biochemistry and psychology) use animals as 'tools' in solving research problems or answering questions about the natural world. The particular use of animals will vary from course to course depending on which research principle or biological concept is being  taught.

### PRODUCTION OF USEFUL BIOLOGICAL AND THERAPEUTIC MATERIALS

Animals also are used in the evaluation of drugs intended for medical or veterinary use, and for the production of useful biological substances. For example, monoclonal antibodies are raised in a variety of animals for use in diagnostic immunological procedures. Similarly, some animals, often horses, are used in the production of anti-venenes used to treat snake bite victims (human and non-human).

### PRODUCT TESTING

Beyond scientific inquiry and education, laboratory animals are used to test consumables in the interests of user safety. Government regulatory agencies[1] often require that such products (chemicals, pharmaceuticals and cosmetics, mainly) be tested before they are released for general use. Animals continue to be used in such testing, including in the following procedures:

- *Acute toxicity tests* consisting of the administration of a single dose of a chemical at a concentration great enough to produce toxic effects and death. An example of such a test is the Lethal Dose 50 ($LD_{50}$) test

---

[1]For example, the 2007 European Union regulation of the Registration, Evaluation, Authorisation and Restriction of Chemicals (REACH). http://echa.europa.eu/regulations/reach

in which 50 per cent of the subjects in an experimental sample are expected to die.

- *Biological screening tests* designed to determine the biological activity of organic compounds in experimental animals.
- *Carcinogenicity tests* where animals, usually rodents, are exposed repeatedly during their life to potential carcinogens (cancer-causing agents).
- *Developmental and reproductive toxicity tests* consisting of several procedures designed to assess the potential of chemicals to induce miscarriages or to cause infertility or birth defects, usually in rodents and rabbits.
- *Eye and skin irritation tests* are designed to determine whether a particular chemical or product will cause irritation on handling or exposure. The notorious Draize test (Draize, Woodward and Calvery 1944), in which rabbits have test substances dripped into one eye (the other acts as a control), is an example.
- *Mutagenicity or genotoxicity tests* are designed to assess whether certain products are capable of causing genetic mutations.
- *Neurotoxicity tests* determine the extent of toxic effects on vertebrate nervous systems. Animal behaviour is observed to detect any lack of coordination, motor disorders, altered learning abilities or gross behavioural changes.
- *Repeated-dose chronic toxicity tests* commonly use rodents to test the effects of repeated exposure (2 weeks to 12 months) to particular chemicals.

# 6    The regulation of experiments

> We all want to be healthy and safe. We want to have the means to
> prevent or cure the health problems and diseases that currently reduce
> the quality of life of millions of people around the world and condemn
> many to an early death ... At the same time most of us would prefer
> animals not to be used to achieve these outcomes, particularly if they
> might be caused pain or harm in the process. The policy-maker's job
> is to find a way of balancing and satisfying each of these conflicting
> societal aspirations in the public interest, as far as current science and
> technologies allow.
>
> *Walsh and Richmond (2005, p. 85)*

LAWS GOVERNING HUMANE USE OF LABORATORY ANIMALS
As already noted, animals are integral to many areas of modern science,
education and product testing. The globalisation of toxicological, pharmaceutical and biomedical research has highlighted a need for an international harmonisation of science quality and best practice in animal
welfare standards through regulation and industry acceptance (Stephens
and Mak 2014; Bayne *et al.* 2015; Burden, Sewell and Chapman 2015;
Fleetwood *et al.* 2015; Medina, Coenen and Kastello 2015). Many nations
now insist on the thorough regulation of all such uses, and this has been
done, albeit in different ways in different countries, with considerable
success (CIOMS and ICLAS 2012).

While it is beyond the scope of this book to review all statutes in all
nations that have laboratory animal welfare legislation, it is worthwhile
to contrast three regulatory approaches: the British centralised government inspectorate system, the US self-regulation system and the
enforced self-regulation systems of Australia and New Zealand that
establish Animal Ethics Committees (AECs). By examining each
system, the extent of legal cover can be explored and the opportunity
for further protection canvassed. Readers interested in a more thorough review of national regulations are referred to comprehensive

discussions elsewhere (Walsh and Richmond 2005; Wolfensohn and Lloyd 2013; Guillén *et al.* 2014; Bayne *et al.* 2015).

The UK *Animals (Scientific Procedures) Act* (1986) is administered through the British Home Office that produces publicly available annual reports that detail aspects of experimentation conducted under the Act (UK Home Office, 2016). The UK Act offers strict protection for all living vertebrates as well as for the common octopus, *Octopus vulgaris*. It controls animal research in the following ways:

1. certification and licensing of researchers and their projects;
2. institutional certification;
3. enforcement through the Animals in Science Regulation Unit inspectorate;
4. the establishment of an independent Animals in Science Committee.

In so doing, it offers laboratory animals four tiers of protection (UK Home Office 2014b). Researchers and other responsible individuals who breach the UK Act are guilty of criminal offences.

### Certification and licensing

Personal and project licences are granted to researchers by the British Home Secretary of State provided they work within an institution that has an Establishment Licence. This licence is given to universities or other research establishments once it has been demonstrated that the institution is a suitable place in which research can be conducted and that the welfare of animals is of concern before, during and after an experiment. Personal licences are given to researchers that can demonstrate, following a period of supervision, an appropriate level of aptitude in specified techniques using designated species. The project licence sets out specifically what can be done as part of any experimental procedure(s), for example collecting blood or drug administration. It limits the severity of experiments (sub-threshold, mild, moderate, severe, non-recovery) based on possible benefits. An experiment with minor costs to an animal in terms of suffering but with substantial potential benefits is more likely to be licensed than a procedure where the opposite is the case (UK Home Office 2014b).

### Establishment Licence

An Establishment Licence is held by a senior individual (e.g. a university vice-chancellor) who is responsible for ensuring that all experimentation falls within the purview of the UK Act. This individual is responsible for appointing named veterinarians and named day-to-day care personnel for projects conducted within the institution. It is his or her responsibility to ensure the welfare of animals held within the institution (UK Home Office 2014b).

### The Animals in Science Regulation Unit inspectorate

The Home Secretary of State appoints inspectors who have three principal duties. First, to consider in detail all licence applications and to advise the Home Secretary how to ensure that only properly justified research is conducted. This includes harm-benefit analyses as a part of each project licence (UK Home Office 2015). Second, to carry out episodic visits to institutions holding Establishment Licences. Inspectors aim to visit all establishments at least once each year to ensure that licence terms and conditions are being met. Finally, as trained medical or veterinary personnel with knowledge of the administration of the UK Act, inspectors are able to give expert advice and assistance to licensees and other personnel (UK Home Office 2014b).

### The Animals in Science Committee

This independent committee has the power to make broad judgements and recommendations to the Home Office about issues in animal experimentation and to advise the government about matters concerning the UK Act. It also advises animal welfare bodies about updates to best practice procedures (UK Home Office 2014b).

### Animal Welfare and Ethical Review Bodies

These four tiers of control emphasise personal responsibility for laboratory animals and the procedures in which they are used, and is generally accepted by those that work within the UK Act as fair and sensible.

The 2013 amendment of the UK *Animals (Scientific Procedures) Act* (1986) resulted in the implementation of institutional Animal Welfare and Ethical Review Bodies. Based on the ethical principles of the 'three Rs' (Russell and Burch 1959) these committees advise staff on matters related to animal husbandry and welfare and promote a 'culture of care' using an evolving document (RSPCA and LASA 2015) which informs best practice.

## AUSTRALIA AND NEW ZEALAND

The regulation of animal experimentation in Australia and New Zealand differs considerably from the UK model. Rather than centralised government administration on a day-to-day basis, these nations operate a form of enforced self-regulation using institutional AECs. Indeed, Australia has no federal legislation that oversees animal experimentation at all. Responsibility for the proper conduct of animal researchers in universities, hospitals, industry and agriculture, currently lies with each state or territory. All states and territories have some form of Prevention of Cruelty to Animals legislation (e.g. Western Australia's *Animal Welfare Act* (2002)). These laws are updated episodically to reflect changes in community concerns. The most recent updates have taken into consideration animals used in experiments and have incorporated adherence to a national code of practice, the *Australian Code for the Care and Use of Animals for Scientific Purposes*. This is an evolving code that was first produced by the Australian National Health and Medical Research Council (NHMRC) in 1969. The *Code* is currently in its eighth edition (NHMRC 2013). It aims to ensure the humane care of non-human vertebrates and cephalopods used for scientific, educational and testing purposes. It does this by:

- emphasising the responsibilities of both the scientists and/or educators using animals and the institutions in which the work is conducted;
- ensuring that the welfare of animals is treated as a priority;
- ensuring that all experimental, testing and teaching procedures are justified within the 'three Rs' principles of Russell and Burch (1959);

- minimising the numbers of animals used, and limiting or avoiding pain or distress;
- actively promoting the use of techniques which replace animal experiments.

The *Code* establishes, and acts as a practical guide for, institutional AECs. Committees consist of at least four people with expertise in separate areas: first, a qualified veterinarian; second, a person with recent experience in animal experimentation; third, a person committed to advancing the welfare of animals (and who is not employed by the institution); fourth, a person independent of the institution who has never had anything to do with animal experimentation.

The regulation of experiments in New Zealand works in a similar way. The New Zealand *Animal Welfare Act* (1999) and *Animal Welfare Amendment Act (No. 2)* (2015) govern what researchers can and cannot do using animals in their care. The New Zealand model differs slightly from its Australian counterpart in that each research institution derives its own Code of Ethical Conduct (New Zealand National Animal Ethics Advisory Committee (NAEAC) 2012), and approval is then sought for each institutional code from NAEAC. No experiments are permitted to proceed prior to approval being gained. At least four people sit on each institutional AEC: one from within the institution and three independent members. One is a veterinarian nominated by the NZ Veterinary Association, one represents a recognised animal welfare group and one is a layperson nominated by a local government body who has no scientific affiliations.

There are presently over 200 AECs in Australia and New Zealand. People who wish to conduct research using animals, whether it be an undergraduate rat or toad dissection or complex surgery involving, say, cats, dogs or kangaroos, must first seek the approval of their AEC. To do this, they must submit a written proposal which includes:

- explicit and achievable aims;
- details of expected benefits flowing from their work;
- details of the vertebrate species to be used;
- consideration of the expected impact on the experimental subjects, and evidence that a cost-benefit analysis, with said impact in mind, has been done;

- evidence that the experimental design is adequate to demonstrate the stated aims;
- details of the ways in which pain and suffering will be alleviated or eliminated before, during and after the planned procedure.

In addition, there is a growing trend for scientists to indicate what alternatives to the use of live animals have been considered during the preparation of AEC applications.

The AEC then considers and approves, modifies or rejects the proposal. With this structure in place, it should not be possible for a poorly thought-out or non-achievable experiment to be conducted. Scientists know that their work will not be permitted to proceed unless they have given thorough consideration to the welfare of animals in their care.

### UNITED STATES OF AMERICA

The US model differs from the British and Australasian systems in that certain vertebrates are currently excluded from protection under government legislation (the Federal *Animal Welfare Act*). This exclusion has led to a number of organisations, both government and non-government, having responsibility for affording protection to all vertebrates used in experiments. Under the *Animal Welfare Act*, animals are defined as:

> any live or dead dog, cat, monkey (nonhuman primate mammal), guinea pig, hamster, rabbit, or such other warm-blooded animal, as the Secretary may determine is being used, or is intended for use, in research, testing, experimentation, or exhibition purposes, or as a pet. (United States Department of Agriculture 2013)

Following amendment in 1971, the Act now specifically excludes:

> (1) birds, rats of the genus *Rattus*, and mice of the genus *Mus*, bred for use in research, (2) horses not used for research purposes, and (3) other farm animals, such as, but not limited to livestock or poultry, used or intended for use as food or fiber or … for improving animal nutrition, breeding, management, or production efficiency, or for improving the quality of food or fiber. (United States Department of Agriculture 2013)

This could be argued as a weakness of the US system, since the majority of US experiments involve an unknown number of purpose-bred rodents that have no legislative protection under the *Animal Welfare Act*. Also excluded by definition are all birds and cold-blooded animals (frogs, toads, salamanders and reptiles) used in research.

In the absence of all-encompassing legislative protection, the US model involves a system of government and non-government organisa-tions all aiming to ensure that the welfare of experimental animals is uppermost. In separate circumstances, each organisation has strong powers to suspend funding, shut down laboratories or withdraw accreditation from research facilities that do not comply with welfare regulations. It is worthwhile to examine the roles of three major insti-tutions in order to understand how the US system protects its research animals from abuse. These are Institutional Animal Care and Use Committees (IACUCs) established by the *Animal Welfare Act*, the National Institutes of Health (NIH) and AAALAC International, a pri-vate organisation that accredits only research laboratories that pursue the highest standards of laboratory animal care.

### Institutional Animal Care and Use Committees

Two broadly complementary federal laws, the *Animal Welfare Act* and the *Health Research Extension Act*, are implemented by regulations stated in the Code of Federal regulations and the Public Health Service (PHS) Policy on Humane Care and Use of Laboratory Animals (National Insti-tutes of Health 2015), respectively. It is the PHS policy, together with the *Animal Welfare Act*, that establishes Institutional Animal Care and Use Committees (IACUCs). Each research facility, whether public or private, has its own committee, and the PHS policy requires each establishment to adhere to the *Guide for the Care and Use of Laboratory Animals* (Eighth edition: National Research Council 2011). IACUCs must have a min-imum of five members to comply with PHS policy, of which at least one member must not be affiliated with the institution and should reflect general community views (National Institutes of Health 2015). In reality, many research facilities have ten or more members on their committee. Each IACUC performs a semi-annual review of the animal care and use programmes and animal house facilities using the National Research

Council *Guide* (2011) as an evaluation base using USDA inspectors. IACUC members also are responsible for reviewing all research protocols prior to their commencement and for reviewing any concerns that may arise during the conduct of research. IACUCs have significant stated responsibilities that require research facilities to provide appropriate veterinary care and pre- and post-operative attention (including the appropriate use of analgesics). An IACUC is authorised to suspend any research that is being conducted outside of the approved protocol.

### The National Institutes of Health

The National Institutes of Health (NIH) funds a significant proportion of animal-based research in the USA. It regulates animal experimentation in both the private and public sectors. The NIH regulations cover all vertebrates including rodents, reptiles and birds. This means that if research is conducted in a university laboratory (or a private laboratory receiving NIH funding), then researchers or laboratories must comply with NIH regulations as well as those established by the *Animal Welfare Act* and administered by IACUCs. Failure to meet strict NIH criteria may result in the suspension of all funding and laboratories being closed down. In many respects the NIH regulations are stronger than those established by the *Animal Welfare Act.*

### AAALAC International

The Association for Assessment and Accreditation of Laboratory Animal Care (AAALAC International) is a private organisation that has conducted a voluntary accreditation programme for laboratories using animals since its inception in 1965. AAALAC International uses performance standards to evaluate and accredit research facilities and institutions. Its regulations are more strict than the NIH and USDA regulations, meaning that research organisations with an AAALAC International 'seal of approval' are of the highest standard when it comes to laboratory animal welfare. The NIH and the National Science Foundation both view AAALAC International accreditation as evidence of exemplary standards of laboratory animal care. This is reflected in the 2015 revision of the PHS policy whereby AAALAC International became recognised as the only accepted accrediting body.

SUMMARY

The British and Australasian systems represent the opposite ends of a regulation spectrum. In the first case, research animals are given a high level of protection based on personal responsibility and criminal sanctions overseen by government representatives. In the latter case, research animals are provided with similar levels of protection through institutional AECs and enforced self-regulation. Each committee has lay and welfare representatives who are in the best position to assert contemporary public opinion about issues in animal experimentation. This means that an experiment with ethical costs approved today may not necessarily be approved tomorrow if popular consensus (reflected on the committee) shifts. In the UK system prior to 1999, Home Office inspectors had acted as 'one-person AECs' (Townsend and Morton 1995), and it is difficult to see how this system could have adequately reflected evolving public attitudes towards animal experimentation in the same way as with Australian and New Zealand AECs. In recognition of this, the Home Secretary of State now requires each research facility to initiate an ethical review process via Animal Welfare and Ethical Review Bodies (UK Home Office 2014b).

The US model is more closely aligned to the Australasian system than to the UK model. Through IACUCs, an acceptable standard of housing and husbandry is enforced, although the *Animal Welfare Act* does not accord legislative protection to all vertebrates. Failure to offer legislative protection to birds, amphibians, reptiles, purpose-bred rodents and livestock used in research has resulted in a complex arrangement whereby government agencies such as the NIH, the PHS and the USDA all have varying powers to control ethical conduct within laboratories. Overlying this system is a private regulatory authority, AAALAC International, that offers accreditation only to facilities where laboratory animal care is of the highest standard.

This mix of public and private regulation may be viewed as a result of the *Animal Welfare Act*'s failure to give legislative protection to all vertebrates. As it stands, though, the complex administrative mix summarised here can be seen to work. Research in public institutions is very highly regulated by the NIH, with strict sanctions enforced in cases where laboratory animal care is lax. In the private sector, marketplace competition may dictate the necessity for companies that conduct (or rely on) animal research and testing to have (or to deal with research institutions that have) AAALAC International accreditation in the first instance to attract further funding, and in the second case to demonstrate a commitment to animal welfare to increasingly informed and concerned consumers.

# 7    Seeking Alternatives

> Perhaps one can see a future where an animal experiment imposes
> no more on the animal than does domestication, and yet can be seen as
> providing a new fulfilment for the animal world – a companionship
> with man in advancing knowledge and, for both, a diminishment of
> future suffering.
>
> *William Paton (1993, p. 230)*

## INTRODUCTION

Despite enormous advancements in research animal welfare, criticism of
animal experimentation remains as vociferous today as it has ever been.
The past 40 years have seen a revitalisation of the animal welfare move-
ment and a consequent proliferation of literature regarding moral, ethical
or regulatory aspects of animal experimentation. After Peter Singer (1975)
and Tom Regan (1983) re-stimulated debate through their professional
interests in the moral status of animals and ethical aspects of animal
research, advocates for the humane treatment of animals, such as Richard Ryder (1975) and Bernard Rollin (1981), chronicled many examples of
modern research of dubious merit and legitimately challenged the value
of results obtained from certain poorly designed experiments.

In the past 40 years in the United Kingdom and elsewhere, there
were unconscionable physical attacks on scientists, their laboratories
and their families by members of an extremist fringe who believed that
the cause of animal welfare could be advanced more quickly by the
publicity their actions generated.

How has the scientific community responded to such challenges?
Some scientists have written books in defence of their disciplines, few
more persuasively than William Paton (1993). Others have been active
in suggesting ways of refining and reducing experimental procedures
with the welfare of laboratory animals in mind. Many researchers have
offered submissions to various government inquiries as legislation has

been drafted or revised to ensure the humane treatment of research animals, or have made valuable contributions to the establishment of effective Animal Ethics Committees (AECs).

Around the world, organisations such as ANZCCART[1], AWIC[2], CCAC[3], FRAME[4], NC3Rs[5] and UFAW[6] provide guidelines for the effective conduct of animal experimentation and up-to-date information on alternatives to the use of sentient animals. In the UK, FRAME, NC3Rs and UFAW regularly inform the scientific and wider community of the availability of new alternatives to the use of animals in experiments via their Web sites. FRAME's principal function is to evaluate techniques for replacing animals in experiments as they are developed and to disseminate such information as widely as possible. This is done primarily through FRAME's Web site and their journal *Alternatives to Laboratory Animals*. NC3Rs promotes the development and dissemination of alternatives underpinned by the 3Rs ethical principles. UFAW produces books on the practical aspects of research animal welfare (e.g. Mellor, Patterson-Kane and Stafford 2009; Hubrecht 2014) and was instrumental in the pioneering of the 'three Rs' (Wickens 2007).

In Australia and New Zealand, a similar role is played by ANZCCART and *ANZCCART News*. In North America, AWIC (in the USA) and CCAC (in Canada) are among the principal institutions that perform similar work.

This chapter examines how such alternatives are being sought, and actively adopted.

### REPLACEMENT, REDUCTION AND REFINEMENT

During the 1950s, UFAW commissioned two scientists, William Russell and Rex Burch, to prepare a manuscript detailing acceptable experimental procedures involving research animals. Their publication, *The Principles*

---

[1]Australian and New Zealand Council for the Care of Animals in Research and Teaching www.adelaide.edu.au/ANZCCART/
[2]Animal Welfare Information Center https://awic.nal.usda.gov/
[3]Canadian Council on Animal Care www.ccac.ca/
[4]Fund for the Replacement of Animals in Medical Experiments www.frame.org.uk
[5]National Centre for the Replacement, Refinement and Reduction of Animals in Research http://nc3rs.org.uk
[6]Universities Federation for Animal Welfare www.ufaw.org.uk/

*of Humane Experimental Technique* (1959), emphasised the need for scientists to appraise their work based on the ethical principles of the 'three Rs'. They recommended that research efforts be directed towards the ultimate replacement of sentient animals in experiments with non-sentient or non-living alternatives at every opportunity. This was recognised as the ideal towards which all researchers should strive (absolute replacement). In the absence of complete replacement, scientists were urged to reduce the number of experiments so that only those considered essential were performed (relative replacement). The number of animals used in such procedures also should be reduced as far as possible, consistent with the requirements of statistical analyses. Finally, scientists were directed to refine experiments to minimise or eliminate completely any suffering involved.

These recommendations have been accepted universally as a corner-stone of modern research practices. Indeed, in some countries, the principles of the 'three Rs' is embodied in legislation. For example, the UK *Animals (Scientific Procedures) Act* (1986) is based on the government decree that

> animal experiments that are unnecessary, use unnecessarily large numbers of animals, or are unnecessarily painful, are undesirable. (cited in FRAME Toxicity Committee 1991, p. 119)

Similarly, the 1986 European Community Directive No. 7.2 insists that

> an experiment shall not be performed if another scientifically satisfactory method of obtaining the result sought, not entailing the use of an animal, is reasonably and practicably available. (cited in FRAME Toxicity Committee 1991, p. 119)

Directive No. 7.3 states:

> When an experiment has to be performed, the choice of species shall be carefully considered and, where necessary, explained to the authority. In a choice between experiments, those which use the minimum number of animals, involve animals with the lowest degree of neurophysiological sensitivity, cause the least pain, suffering, distress or lasting harm and which are most likely to provide satisfactory results shall be selected. (Balls 1990, p. 227)

In toxicity testing, regulatory organisations and statutory authorities provide policy directions that integrate the 'three Rs' principles (e.g. the EU REACH[7] programme and JRC Science and Policy Reports[8], and the USA National Research Council 2007).

There is little doubt that all concerned with the welfare of animals see the notion of the 'three Rs' as worthy. Some would argue, however, that progress towards alternatives is inexorably slow, and much research should be suspended until alternatives are available. Others argue that we neglect vital research while alternatives are sought. Still others argue a middle path where we actively encourage the search for alternatives while maintaining essential and humanely conducted research.

## ALTERNATIVES TO NON-HUMAN VERTEBRATES IN SCIENTIFIC RESEARCH

### Definitions

In each of the areas of scientific research described in Chapter 5, there is a wide scope for the application of alternatives encompassing the 'three Rs' (National Research Council 2007). The success of such an approach to the reform of modern animal experimentation is that it does not impede the fundamental aims of scientific endeavour. Rather, it presents an essentially pro-science ideal which challenges researchers to develop affordable and ethically superior experimental methods (Gauthier and Griffin 2005).

For the purposes of this discussion, alternatives to animal experiments can be usefully defined (after Smyth 1978) as:

> procedures which can completely replace the need for animal experiments, reduce the number of animals required, or diminish the amount of pain or distress suffered by the animals in meeting the essential needs of [humans] and other animals.

This is a definition which has gained wide acceptance worldwide (but see Stephens and Mak 2014; Tannenbaum and Bennett 2015 for various points of view).

---

[7] http://echa.europa.eu/regulations/reach
[8] E.g. EU JRC 2014. *EURL ECVAM strategy to replace, reduce and refine the use of animals in the assessment of acute mammalian systemic toxicity.*

The examples I use below are widely known and, for the most part, proven by years of successful use. They serve to illustrate the principles of the 'three Rs'. The search for alternatives is ongoing, and readers are referred to the NORINA[9] database for updated versions available on a suite of media and Web-based packages, or alternatives specific to their areas of interest.

### Replacement alternatives

Replacement alternatives eliminate the use of vertebrates in particular experiments. Such methods can be classified into several categories:

1. the use of less-sentient (or non-sentient) organisms (invertebrates and microorganisms);
2. the use of *in vitro* techniques;
3. the use of *in silico* techniques;
4. human studies.

#### The use of less-sentient (or non- sentient) organisms

The presence in biological systems of broadly applicable physiological and anatomical generalisations makes it possible to substitute non-sentient life forms in experiments which might otherwise involve vertebrates. This is perhaps best illustrated by the principle of 'unity in diversity' (National Research Council 1985). Despite myriad differences between animal species, unity is evident based upon common anatomical features and the general similarity of cell function and development pathways. For example, the process of early embryonic development in all vertebrates follows the same pathway. Every vertebrate, whether a fish or a human, grows from a blastula stage and follows a genetically programmed development that includes the formation of ectodermal, mesodermal and endodermal cells. Molecular biology offers further evidence of similarities between species – the genetic code applies to all microorganisms, plants and animals (National Research Council 1988). If invertebrates and early-stage vertebrate embryos, as well as plants, bacteria and other microorganisms,

[9]Norwegian Reference Centre for Laboratory Animal Science and Alternatives http:// oslovet.norecopa.no/fag.aspx?fag=57

all show common cellular and biochemical traits, then they all offer the opportunity for development as alternatives to using fully developed vertebrates in experimentation.

*Examples*
- An alternative to the use of mammals in some experiments is a simple test that uses the coelenterate *Hydra* to detect chemicals that may produce foetal abnormalities (teratogens). This procedure is based on the observation that vertebrate teratogens also impede the normal development of *Hydra* (Yum *et al.* 2014).
- Some invertebrates offer widespread alternatives for students in primary and secondary education. Organisms such as flatworms, earthworms, some molluscs, insects and crustaceans all may be substituted for vertebrates as simple systems of sophisticated biological phenomena.

Such organisms are not necessarily the ones with which students normally show a great deal of empathy (certain mammals generally elicit stronger bonds). However, it is a relatively simple task for teachers to emphasise common links between humans and all other creatures, or to explain why a 'lower' species is being used in preference to a 'higher' one.

### The use of in vitro techniques

*In vitro* (in-glass) methods afford researchers the opportunity to study many physiological systems outside the body (Davies 2012a). Currently, technology is available which permits the culturing of cells and tissues (see Daston *et al.* 2015), the maintenance of organs and organ slices in nutrient media (see Wick *et al.* 2015) and organ-on-a-chip biomimicry (see Zheng *et al.* 2016). Such techniques have other advantages over *in vivo* methods. Cells and tissues can be studied in an isolated environment, away from the influence of integrated physiological systems. The influence of such systems may then be mimicked under controlled conditions in further experiments. Another obvious advantage is that drugs can be tested on tissue derived from humans, thereby obviating the need for extrapolation from an animal model to the human condition.

In many countries, institutional AECs require researchers to demonstrate that they have sought alternatives to the use of vertebrates. Information about *in vitro* techniques are made readily available to researchers through a suite of internet sites and databases (e.g. Hakkinen and Green 2002; Zhu *et al.* 2014).

*Examples*
- Cell, tissue or organ chips or cultures can be used to test potentially toxic chemicals in rigidly controlled trials. Cultured cells can be observed microscopically while a suspected toxin is added. Rather than administering a drug that is thought to cause heart palpitations in vertebrates to a group of white mice, researchers can simply record changes in the beating of cultured heart cells *in vitro* in response to the drug.
- In the pharmaceutical industry and in toxicological research, tissue culture techniques have been used to screen potential anti-viral agents and to assess damage to DNA (e.g. Cordelli *et al.* 2007; National Research Council 2007; Stephens and Mak 2014). Rather than inoculate vertebrates (usually mice) with each test substance, cell and organ chips or cultures may be utilised (Zheng *et al.* 2016).
- Skin irritation tests using reconstructed human epidermis (Poumay and Coquette 2007; Jung *et al.* 2014; Miles *et al.* 2014) offer an *in vitro* alternative to chemical and cosmetic testing using guinea pigs and rabbits.

### The use of in silico *techniques*

Non-biological, or *in silico*, alternatives to experiments using vertebrates currently include mathematical modelling, computer simulation and the use of audiovisual techniques for education and training. Mathematical modelling is currently being used in the active designing of pharmaceuticals for specific purposes, the modelling of biochemical, toxicological and physiological processes, and the predictive modelling known as QSAR modelling. Quantitative structure-activity relationships (QSAR) are modelled to predict potential toxic activity of chemical compounds based on molecular structure. By examining the physical parameters of molecules in a certain chemical compound, QSAR modelling enables predictions to be made about the toxicity of new compounds containing similar molecules. The use of the Draize rabbit eye irritation test (see Chapter 5) has been greatly reduced by the application of QSARs (e.g. Abraham *et al.* 2003, Gerner, Liebsch and Spielmann 2005; Kar and Roy 2014).

Mathematical models also may be generated to predict the outcome of certain research pathways. Used in this way, such models can reduce unnecessary and wasteful research, thereby saving time, money and experimental subjects.

Computer simulation offers many opportunities for reducing the numbers of procedures involving vertebrates in education and training.

*Examples*

- *Sniffy the Virtual Rat*[10] and *Rat Dissection for iPad*[11] are excellent examples of the types of alternatives to classroom dissection and undergraduate animal behaviour experiments accessible through the NORINA internet site. *Sniffy the Virtual Rat* is an interactive programme that provides students with a virtual Skinner Box in which simulated animal behaviours can be observed. With apps such as *Rat Dissection for iPad*, rather than dissecting a rat bred and purchased for undergraduate use, students can simulate a dissection in a non-intimidatory way, at their own pace. Functional anatomy is emphasised with high-resolution imaging as the student conducts a simulated dissection. *The Digital Frog*[12] programme offers similar features as well as incorporating information on behaviour, life cycle and ecology.
- Sophisticated simulations such as *Anatomy and Physiology Revealed*[13] continue to offer medical and physiology students alternative methods of coming to grips with the interactive nature of brain, heart and circulatory function and fluid physiology. *Pictures Instead*

[10]http://oslovet.veths.no/produkt.aspx?produkt=4582
[11]http://oslovet.norecopa.no/produkt.aspx?produkt=9119
[12]http://oslovet.norecopa.no/produkt.aspx?produkt=4735
[13]http://oslovet.norecopa.no/produkt.aspx?produkt=4772

*of Animals*[14] is a downloadable compilation of digital images which illustrate adverse pharmaceutical reactions.

It is unlikely that simulations will completely replace the need for actual dissections or experiments. However, today many undergraduate science students do not follow a career in veterinary or physiological research where a case might be made that it is more important that students are trained with animals.

Video presentations offer students a wide range of non-experimental options in learning. Audiovisual aids may demonstrate surgical technique or teach correct procedures for handling live animals. Although they cannot offer 'hands-on' experience, some particularly sophisticated videos are available for download, e.g. the Norwegian School of Veterinary Science's *Handling and Basic Techniques*[15].

The extension of non-biological alternatives has also seen the widespread use of computer-linked mannequins to provide sophisticated simulations. An early example, *Resusci-Dog*, was a simulator developed at Cornell University, New York, for veterinary students. It was the equivalent of the human mannequins used in the training of resuscitation techniques, but was driven by microprocessors. It could simulate a femoral artery pulse and could be used for cardiac massage. It was reported that *Resusci-Dog* replaced as many as 100 dogs previously used by students each year at Cornell University (US Congress, Office of Technology Assessment 1986).

More modern mannequins such as the feline *Critical Care Fluffy*[16] continue to provide students with improved non-animal alternatives for veterinary training.

Virtual reality computer simulation offers users an opportunity to 'perform' experiments such as laparoscopies without the need for a patient. By connecting a laparoscope to a virtual reality generator, images of what a surgeon 'sees' as he or she 'enters' a body are produced. Such technology is still in its infancy but currently holds the potential to outstrip other simulation methods in the near future.

[14]http://oslovet.norecopa.no/produkt.aspx?produkt=89
[15]http://oslovet.norecopa.no/produkt.aspx?produkt=5743
[16]http://oslovet.norecopa.no/produkt.aspx?produkt=5233

*Human studies*

A final replacement alternative worthy of consideration is the use of humans rather than other vertebrates. Tissues derived from humans *post mortem* are able to be used for many purposes. Additionally, human placentae can be used, for example, as a source of cells for tissue culture, or in the training of microsurgical techniques (US Congress, Office of Technology Assessment 1986).

The delivery to humans of microdoses of pharmaceuticals that are in the early stages of development also holds promise as a method that may eliminate the need for some drug testing using animal models (Lappin, Noveck and Burt 2013).

Research has also been conducted using human volunteers. Under the 1975 Tokyo Amendment to the 1964 Helsinki Declaration (Tyebkhan 2003), volunteers consent to a particular experiment after being informed of specific procedures and the inherent risks. Students of medicine, physiology and psychology are often involved in non-invasive experiments where they use one another as 'guinea pigs'. In industry and cosmetics testing, products with the potential for irritancy have been trialled on volunteers rather than on non-humans (e.g. Benassi, Bertazzoni and Seidenari 1999; Tsunoda *et al.* 2014).

The development of new pharmaceutical agents currently involves exhaustive testing using *in vitro* techniques, non-human vertebrates and, ultimately, human testing. Could we not move simply from *in vitro* development to testing on volunteers, eliminating the need for research animal testing? The response to such a question rests entirely on the degree of risk society as a whole is prepared to take. It is worthwhile to consider the development of one drug, thalidomide, to assist in forming an opinion.

*The tragedy of thalidomide* Thalidomide caused birth defects in children in the early 1960s after it had been prescribed to women to alleviate morning sickness early in pregnancy. It was first developed in Europe as a sedative in the mid-1950s. The manufacturer described it as structurally analogous to barbiturates, although its method of action was never investigated (National Health and Medical Research Council 1990). Following testing in rodents, the company distributed thalidomide to doctors, claiming it to be a rapid-acting, long-lasting sedative. No teratogenicity studies were conducted. Early reports of side effects involving the central nervous system and a general lack of tolerance to the prescribed dose rates were ignored and, in 1957, the manufacturer released the drug on the general non-prescription market in an influenza mixture (National Health and Medical Research Council 1990). In 1960, there was a spate of abnormal births from mothers who had taken thalidomide early in pregnancy. Children were born with digestive tract abnormalities and with incompletely developed or absent limbs.

Thalidomide was withdrawn from sale in October 1961. Intensive testing for teratogenicity using many animal species yielded markedly variable results. Pregnant guinea pigs and mice which had been dosed with thalidomide did not give birth to abnormal offspring. Rats of different strains showed varying sensitivity to thalidomide. Not all strains were sensitive, and those which were reabsorbed abnormal fetuses, thus masking the results of experiments designed to produce the malformed young. Dogs did not show gross abnormalities, although some puppies were born with necrotic tail tips and first toes. It was not until 1962 that birth defects similar to those seen in humans were found in laboratory animals. Pregnant New Zealand White rabbits dosed with thalidomide gave birth to fewer young, with increased rates of stillbirth and reduction deformities. Testing using macaques, rhesus monkeys and marmosets showed birth abnormalities similar to those seen in human babies (National Health and Medical Research Council 1990).

What we know now, but did not know then, is that the timing during pregnancy of the administration of a drug in a teratogenicity trial is critical. Different species have different gestation lengths, and teratogenicity effects are highly dependent on the stage of pregnancy at which a drug is given.

The tragedy of thalidomide has been used to argue both for and against the use of drug testing on non-human animals. Opponents claim that the physiologies of animals used for drug testing are sufficiently different from human physiology for such testing to be essentially useless. Proponents of drug testing using laboratory animals use the same example of thalidomide to argue that current levels of animal use should be maintained to ensure that such a tragedy can never occur again.

### Reduction alternatives

There are powerful ethical reasons for reducing the numbers of vertebrates used in experiments. Morally, it is our duty to limit any distress caused to laboratory animals during confinement or experimentation. The onus is on every researcher to justify each proposed action as the *exclusive* means to their desired end, to use fewer sentient animals, animals of lesser sentience, and to employ less painful procedures at every opportunity.

There are several tried and tested methods for reducing numbers of research animals. These include pooling available resources, using the appropriate statistical techniques and not repeating experiments unnecessarily. Well-organised research establishments hold regular seminars so that scientists are constantly kept abreast of work being conducted in other departments. Regular communication between scientists provides opportunities for pooling of resources. It makes good sense for researchers to collaborate whenever possible and to arrange for the simultaneous use of animals in more than one project. For example, if an animal has been bred or purchased for the periodic collection of blood or for tissue biopsy, it can then be used prior to euthanasia for the collection of cells for culture, or its organs may be used *post mortem* in histological investigations. If a wild animal is captured for experimentation and is to be euthanased at the end of the research, the carcass ought to be given, whenever possible, to a museum so that a taxidermist can prepare it for educative purposes. Obviously, there are many instances when the sharing of laboratory animals is not feasible, but it must be part of the modern training process that researchers constantly seek novel ways to lower the number of animals used in science.

*Unnecessary* repetition of experiments is best avoided by adhering to long-established scientific procedures including the thorough searching of technical literature, scientific journals and online databases, peer review prior to experimentation and the *rapid* publication of results. By reviewing one's topic thoroughly, it may be found that a particular experiment has already been conducted elsewhere, or previous research can assist in the modification of proposed research. Modern search filters and data-mining programmes are facilitating this (e.g. Hooijmans *et al.* 2010; Zhang, Hsieh and Zhu 2014).

Peer review will aid in minimising the number of animals used in each procedure by directing inexperienced researchers to the appropriate statistical method when designing their experiments (see, for example, *Experimental Design*[17], a computer program which assists researchers to design more effective experiments).

The onus is on competent researchers to make available as much information as possible about the experiments they have conducted when they publish in the scientific literature. For example, information about the number and species/strain of animal used (Kilkenny *et al.* 2009), and details of all animal handling methods ought to be given (Hoggatt *et al.* 2016; Jackson *et al.* 2016). To this end, guidelines that assist researchers about what information to report have been endorsed as best practice by journal editors worldwide (e.g. CONSORT[18] (Plint *et al.* 2006) and ARRIVE[19] (Kilkenny *et al.* 2010)).

Many experiments must be repeated. In some instances, earlier results need to be checked for accuracy – particularly when new models or techniques are being developed. Reproducibility is a cornerstone of the scientific method. It is being shown increasingly in some fields that small, sometimes trivial differences in the conditions under which an experiment is conducted can produce vastly different results. For example, differences in the methods of blood collection from mice are now known to affect numerous blood parameters significantly (Hoggatt *et al.* 2016). We now know, too, that many physiological systems are affected markedly by photoperiod. An experiment conducted in the morning may yield completely different results from one performed in the afternoon. It is now being discovered that in certain circumstances long-regarded 'facts' are by no means universal and may hold only under specific conditions (Calisi and Bentley 2009). This has important implications for animal researchers. It is critical that any variation inherent in a system be taken into consideration when designing an experiment.

Competent scientists recognise that their careers depend on their ability to attract research funds and then to use these funds efficiently in pursuit

---

[17]www.sheffbp.co.uk/products/experdis.htm
[18]Consolidated Standards of Reporting Trials
[19]Animals in Research: Reporting *In Vivo* Experiments

of their goals. To this end, a great deal of thought must be given to the design of any experiment. No granting body is going to be interested in awarding financial or other resources to researchers who have not given thorough consideration to their proposed research. This is especially relevant in projects where animals are to be used: the repercussions of a 'slap happy' approach to research may be far-reaching.

Research scientists must formulate their grant application with *specific* aims in mind. Applicants will be given short shrift by referees acting on behalf of a funding body if little thought is evident in this facet of experimental design. Modern experimentation demands that research aims be both *achievable* and *worthwhile*. In designing any experiment which involves animals, the first question to be addressed must be: Is this experiment necessary? A thorough review of the scientific literature may often reveal similar work conducted elsewhere. Such a finding may call into question the relevance of the experimental aims, in which case a researcher must be prepared to return to the drawing board. It is no longer acceptable that scientists expend their time (and their subjects' lives) conducting ill-conceived or already completed experiments.

Having decided that a particular project has achievable aims, the next step is to justify the research in terms of perceived benefits. Deciding whether the entire exercise is worthwhile is necessarily a subjective assessment. No one can be completely sure of the outcomes of an experiment until it has been performed. Consequently, several factors must be taken into account when assessing an experiment's relative merits.

Smith and Boyd (1991) proposed criteria by which a project's aims ought to be judged. First, an experiment will be deemed worthwhile if it has *potential* economic, educational, scientific and/or social value. Second, one must assess the *likelihood* that any predicted benefit will be realised. A third criterion urges a review of the *quality* of the experiment in relation to its scientific method and the applicability of the proposed techniques. This criterion is possibly the most important one as it deals with the methods which are to be used to realise an experiment's aims. Smith and Boyd (1991) suggested that researchers ought to assess their proposed methods in several ways.

- Are the methods relevant in answering a particular scientific question?
- Is it necessary to use animals at all?
- If so, is the species, and number of individuals of that species, appropriate?
- Is it necessary to use procedures of the proposed severity?
- Has the amount of information to be obtained from each animal been maximised, subject to welfare restraints?
- Are the research facilities, scientists and technicians of sufficient quality for the work to be completed successfully?

To this list I would also add:

- Is veterinary advice available, and has the use of anaesthetics and analgesics been given appropriate consideration?

Anyone closely associated with a particular research project may review their proposed experiment with the above questions in mind and genuinely believe that all have been answered satisfactorily. It is at this point that consultation with colleagues not immediately associated with the proposed research is important. Peer review, properly conducted, provides an effective method of ensuring that most aspects of experimental design are carried out correctly. Colleagues will highlight obvious flaws in reasoning and suggest alternatives. Many research institutions now insist that a thorough peer review process is conducted before any scientist applies for research funding. This necessarily includes in-house seminars for a free exchange of ideas with other scientists and an opportunity for the suggestion of improvements. It also includes mandatory consultation with statisticians to ensure that both the planning and proposed analyses of results are acceptable. Statistical techniques must be used in order to differentiate between the effects of a particular experimental procedure and random variation. A correctly designed experiment will ensure that a researcher can be confident that any results obtained are in response to an experimental manipulation rather than any variability in the system.

An equally important duty of the statistician is to assist in determining how many animals ought to be used for a given procedure. Obviously, it is not appropriate from an ethical standpoint to have too many individuals for each procedure. However, scientists, in their desire to reduce the number of individuals to be used in a proposed experiment, may well weaken their design by having too *few* individuals. This can be as wasteful as having too many, because the experiment will prove statistically inconclusive and have to be repeated to augment the data. A statistician can best determine the appropriate number of animals and treatments to be used to answer a specific question; it is important that all scientists recognise that the contribution of the statistician is indispensable in modern research (see Parker and Browne 2014 for a comprehensive review).

Once an experiment has been designed to the satisfaction of the investigators and their peers (including statisticians), any proposal involving experiments on sentient animals is either submitted to a government representative (e.g. in the United Kingdom) or to an Animal Ethics Committee (AEC). In the countries where they have been established, AECs operate on the basis that human welfare has precedence over the welfare of animals, but that the use of non-humans for scientific purposes is strictly conditional. Generally speaking, AEC and government guidelines for evaluating proposals make clear that animals should be used only to obtain important information in essential experiments, that all animals used in experiments are treated with respect, and that the welfare of research animals before, during and after experimentation is given careful consideration. With such stipulations in mind, each representative, whether he or she is a British Home Office inspector or an American IACUC member, must balance the potential gains which may accrue beyond an experiment with the inherent costs in terms of distress, poor health or pain and/or suffering of the experimental subjects. It is the responsibility of every AEC member to sanction an experiment only when there have been genuine and thorough attempts by the researcher to minimise suffering and when the potential benefits outweigh inherent costs to animals associated with husbandry, housing, experimentation and post-operative conditions.

### Refinement alternatives

The third alternative principle is refinement – the modification, to minimise animal suffering, of procedures which must involve sentient animals. Again, it is every researcher's responsibility to answer several questions prior to commencing an experiment. Having first ascertained that the problem is worth solving and that the animal proposed for use is the best model, questions of refinement need to be addressed. Will the experimental subjects be housed adequately? Must the animals be conscious for the procedure? Does each researcher have the appropriate skills to conduct each procedure humanely? These and other considerations must be given careful thought as part of an 'alternatives' strategy.

A thorough knowledge of the relevant literature is essential. Many professional societies and policy makers issue guidelines for the use of vertebrates in research, and scientists should make themselves familiar with such publications (see, for example, Association for the Study of Animal Behaviour 2012; OECD 2012; Use of Fishes in Research Committee 2013; Hodgson and Koh 2016; Sikes et al. 2016). Other refinement techniques include the following:

1. improved animal husbandry, which reduces the stress of handling (gentling) and utilises more sympathetic environmental conditions for confining animals (enrichment);
2. the use of anaesthesia during all surgical procedures and analgesia in postoperative care to alleviate pain;
3. the use of alternative methods of drug and product testing where the severity of endpoints in experiments is reduced.

### Improved animal husbandry and enrichment

Much of the distress which laboratory animals or wild animals held in captivity may endure might not involve actual physical pain. Anxiety, altered physiology due to inadequate exercise or the physiological responses of animals to confinement and handling must all be given due consideration (Wolfensohn and Lloyd 2013; Sikes and Bryan 2015). Environmental conditions within animal houses and laboratories vary enormously. Changes in temperature, humidity, light regime and noise intensity all may contribute to environmental stress. Similarly, the level of animal husbandry may vary during the working week and on weekends, or the standards of diet, bedding, cage cleaning and technical and gentling skills of animal house attendants may fluctuate. All of these factors may cause detectable physiological responses to stress that may lead to aberrant results in many experiments. *Stress* is defined here, after Hungarian physiologist Hans Selye (1975, p. 324), as 'the state manifested by a specific syndrome which consists of all non-specifically induced changes within a biological system.' Anything which produces a state of stress, Selye termed a *stressor*. This definition was later modified to include not only harmful stimuli but also stimuli *perceived* to be harmful (Selye 1976).

The importance of psychological variables in determining the extent of the physiological effects of stressors is well known. Today, stress research emphasises a relationship between physiology and behaviour. For example, an animal exposed to a novel environment is not necessarily in any danger *per se*. Nevertheless, that animal will respond with behavioural changes, increased heart rate and corticosteroid hormone secretion (Moberg 2000). These reactions are indicative of a stress response, even though a new environment does not represent an actual threat to the maintenance of a homeostatic state.

The influence of an individual's perception of a stressor, rather than the stressor itself, is well known. Exposure of laboratory animals to identical physical stressors (e.g. electric shock) with different psychological components (e.g. some individuals given warning buzzers prior to the electric shocks) can result in a different development rate of stomach ulceration – a common pathological symptom of stress. Those individuals which were warned prior to being shocked tended to develop stress ulcers at an increased rate (Weiss 1972).

Merely having their cages moved by an animal house attendant, something which is done daily as cages and rooms are cleaned, has been found to be a sufficient enough stressor to alter measured blood characteristics associated with stress and shock in some strains of laboratory rats (Gärtner *et al.* 1980; Balcombe, Barnard and Sandusky 2004).

Clearly, anxiety and emotional arousal are factors that can determine the extent of a physiological stress response and must be taken into account in all experiments involving sentient animals. Environmental enrichment, which provides animals with physical and mental stimulation as a part of their captive environment, is an extremely important way of reducing the risks associated with stress and enhancing the validity of the research results (Bayne and Würbel 2014). To this end, numerous internet databases exist to which contributions can be made by interested parties to facilitate the uptake or modification of animal housing techniques that promote well-being (Baumans et al. 2007). One example of how environmental enrichment has been widely promoted and adopted involves colonies of captive-bred and wild-caught primates (National Institutes of Health 2005; National Centre for the Replacement Refinement and Reduction of Animals in Research 2006). Primate species including marmosets, macaques and rhesus monkeys are used in biomedical research and for safety testing of pharmaceuticals. Such species are intelligent and highly mobile and require social interactions and constant mental and physical stimulation. Provision of pair housing, group housing and a constant supply of novel items to investigate all form vital parts of an enriched environment (Baker and Dettmer 2016).

The adjustment of wild animals to confinement is also relevant to almost all behavioural or physiological studies involving experimentation. Similarly, any long-term studies of the ecology and behaviour of free-living wildlife must take into account any effects of short-term or prolonged physiological responses to capture when the study involves trapping and handling (Monamy and Gott 2001; Lindsjö, Fahlman and Törnqvist 2016). It has been long known that prior to experimentation, even highly domesticated species, such as laboratory rats, require extensive periods of acclimation (Grant et al. 1971). It is safe to assume that the same must apply to wild animals in captivity, particularly if a species shows a susceptibility to capture or confinement stress. A great deal of information has been obtained on the behaviour and physiology of wild animals from captive colonies, and the question arises whether such information is pertinent to the species involved or to the conditions in which the animals were held.

Environmental stress can be reduced in animal houses by ensuring

- appropriate lighting, temperature and humidity control;
- that noise (including ultrasound levels) is kept to an absolute minimum;

- adequate air conditioning to stop the build-up of noxious gases (e.g. ammonia), and to prevent odours from one species (e.g. dogs) from being detected by another species that may be distressed if such odours were detected (e.g. rabbits).

A well-run animal housing facility simply does not have slamming doors, curious and noisy visitors, or unprofessional workers. Ideally, senior staff ought to have veterinary skills and the ability to liaise with research staff to ensure that they are giving due consideration to what happens to their animals before *and* after they have been used in an experiment.

In an important declaration, the British Institute of Medical Ethics multi-disciplinary working party on animal welfare stated:

> The manner in which laboratory animals are housed and cared for is of utmost importance in determining the overall quality of their lives. Researchers should take particular care for the conditions under which the animals they use are maintained; and housing and husbandry conditions should be taken into account when assessing the overall costs of a particular piece of research. Where possible, more natural or enriched environments should be provided, so that the animals can carry out more of their natural behaviour patterns and fulfil their psychological needs. (Smith and Boyd 1991, p. 332)

Carefully controlled husbandry practices such as promoting positive animal welfare states (Mellor 2015a), providing domestic animals with an opportunity to interact with humans (Cloutier, Panksepp and Newberry 2012) or keeping wild animals in conditions where inter-species interactions are minimal will result in healthier animals. The results of any experiments using such animals are likely to be more accurate than in procedures where poorly educated or uncaring researchers have not had the welfare of their animals uppermost in their minds (see Bayne and Würbel 2014). Increasingly, too, re-homing of healthy farm animals after they have been used in certain experiments is being encouraged as part of refinement protocols.

### The use of anaesthesia and analgesia

*The perception of pain* The perception of pain has been the subject of furious debate (see, for example, Rutherford 2002; National Research

Council 2008; Whittaker and Howarth 2014). What is pain? We would all agree that, under most circumstances, when we cut ourselves, it hurts. But how do you describe what you are feeling to someone else? Pain may be of short or long duration, and can range, subjectively, from mild to severe in intensity. Pain specialists have evaluated pain in humans and emphasise two distinct aspects – stimulus and perception.

The important aspect to recognise is the interconnection of two components: *nociception* – the detection and signalling of a noxious stimulus; and the conscious *recognition* of pain derived from that stimulus. Beyond the pain tolerance threshold is *suffering*: 'the affective, behavioural or emotional response to the pain' (Rose and Adams 1989). It is the subjectivity inherent in any perception of a noxious stimulus, the variability in pain tolerance thresholds and the differing behavioural or emotional responses to pain that make it so difficult to define. Indeed, it may be argued that it is not possible to describe to another the pain one is feeling, or to comprehend another person's misery.

Does the same apply to non-human beings? Do they respond to noxious stimuli differently? As individuals? As species? If so, how do individuals communicate their distress? Are we sufficiently sensitive to detect it?

Philosophers and scientists have wrestled with these questions in an effort to reach consensus on definitions of intra-species and inter-species pain perception (see Sneddon *et al.* 2014). We have used some non-human species to model pain in humans because the anatomical and chemical pathways by which pain is perceived in these non-humans have been shown to be similar to those in humans (Morton and Griffiths 1985). Is it not logical, then, to reverse the situation and assume that such non-humans perceive pain as we do?

In the absence of objectivity, certain assumptions about pain perception and communication in non-humans have been made. Smith and Boyd (1991) suggested that a non-human being's capacity to experience pain could be tested in two ways. First, does a species have similar anatomical, biochemical and physiological mechanisms 'to those which in a human are known to be correlated with such experiences?' Second, 'does the animal perform in similar ways to humans who are believed to be suffering?' (Smith and Boyd 1991, p. 46). In the absence of definitive answers to either of these questions, a pragmatic approach can be adopted, based on two assumptions. First, we accept philosopher Stephen Clark's (1984, p. 42) simple observation that 'pain is painful' as a working definition of what constitutes pain. Second, although some differences undoubtedly exist between human and non-human beings, conditions that are perceived as painful in humans should be assumed to be perceived as painful in other animals. This assumption formed the basis for the cautious suggestion put forward by Kitchell and Erickson (1983, p. viii):

> When considering pain in animals, analogies must be drawn between human and animal anatomy, physiology and behaviour. Knowledge about pain in animals remains inferential however, and neglect of the probabilistic nature of pain perception in animals leads to anthropomorphism. On the other hand, overemphasis on the uncertainty of our knowledge about pain perception in animals, which leads to a denial that pain perception exists in animals, is logically as well as empirically unfounded. That tacit assumption is that stimuli are noxious and strong enough to give rise to the perception of pain in animals if the stimuli are detected as pain by human beings, if they at least approach or exceed tissue-damaging proportions, and if they produce escape behaviour in animals.

*The recognition and alleviation of pain* Pain and distress in animal subjects occur in two main branches of scientific work. The first branch comprises studies that investigate the nature of pain itself. In such procedures, the anatomical, behavioural, chemical and physiological mechanisms associated with pain are monitored, with the ultimate aim being the prevention, reduction or treatment of pain in human and non-human animals (Graham 2016). The testing of analgesic drugs can also result in some pain as part of an experimental trial. To minimise this, novel practices have emerged. For example, Curtright *et al.* (2015) used zebrafish larvae to measure the analgesic properties of a variety of chemicals. They set up aquaria with discrete temperature zones (too hot, too cold, just right) and measured the time spent in each zone by groups of fish, assuming that the analgesic properties of any chemicals that they then added would mean that the fish would swim in hotter and/or colder zones for longer.

The second branch covers all other kinds of animal experimentation where pain is a completely unintended side effect which may cloud the results being sought. Despite the difficulties associated with an object-ive definition of pain, it is important to be able to recognise signs that an animal is in pain. A significant paper published in the British journal *Veterinary Record* in April 1985 first detailed ways in which pain, distress and discomfort could be recognised in animals used in experiments (Morton and Griffiths 1985). Researchers were urged to watch for changes in appearance, dietary intake and behaviour, as well as in clinical signs such as altered heart rate, abnormal breathing or muscle twitching. It is important that more than one criterion be used when assessing pain or distress (Wolfensohn and Lloyd 2013). For example, an animal may appear outwardly to be behaving quite normally but may be losing weight rapidly. The principle to be applied here is – *know your animal*. Learn to recognise symptoms which may indicate that an animal is in pain. These might include the following (US Congress, Office of Technology Assessment 1986; Wolfensohn and Lloyd 2013):

- Impaired activity – for example an individual may remain immobile in its cage.
- Personality changes such as increased aggression.
- Restlessness, where an animal cannot stay in the one position and is constantly getting up and lying down.
- Changes in the rate of intake of food or water.
- Abnormal vocalisation.
- Abnormal posture.
- Self-mutilation.

If it is suspected that an animal is in pain, veterinary advice must be sought, and it is the moral (and in many countries, legal) obligation of every researcher to supply pain relief where applicable. This can be done in three ways; *tranquillising, anaesthetising* or administering an *analgesic*. Tranquillisers have calming effects, reducing anxiety and tension. They lower the level of consciousness but do not offer pain relief. They are particularly suitable in preventing animals struggling while being handled or measured, or for reducing the distress sometimes associated with confinement.

Anaesthetics eliminate the sensation of pain, with varying effects on consciousness. Topical and local anaesthetics do not alter consciousness to the same degree as general anaesthesia. Topical anaesthetics (usually ointments) are used in the treatment of minor injuries; local anaesthetics are used in minor surgery; general anaesthetics render an animal completely unconscious, usually while surgery is conducted. In all cases where an anaesthetic is used, postoperative observation is essential to ensure that anaesthetised areas are not damaged because of a patient's loss of sensation.

Analgesics relieve pain without altering consciousness. They are used most frequently following surgery. In *all* cases where it is likely that pain is perceived, analgesics must be given.

*Humane endpoints*

Increasing attention is being given to research protocols to determine whether more humane endpoints (the point at which an experiment is deemed to be over) ought to be applied (Morton 2000; Franco, Correa-Neves and Olsson 2012; Ashall and Millar 2014). Pre-lethal and, ideally, pre-painful endpoints are constantly sought in toxicity trials and drugs testing, where controversial procedures such as the Draize eye instillation test and the $LD_{50}$ test have been used. Promising alternatives are being developed, including a range of *in vitro* techniques to replace carcinogenicity and irritancy tests (Stephens and Mak 2014). In experiments where tumours are deliberately induced in animals, the severity of an endpoint can be minimised by limiting the size to which the tumour is permitted to grow. Similarly, in certain animal models of disease or in radiation studies, euthanasia ought to be used rather than letting an animal die slowly or painfully.

Alternatives such as those described above point to the future direction of animal experimentation. It is the responsibility of all researchers to modify their techniques to incorporate, where possible, existing alternatives, and to seek novel alternative methods which will continue the reform of animal experimentation.

# 8    A future without animal experimentation?

> In relative replacement, animals are still required, though in actual
> experiment they are exposed, probably or certainly, to no distress at all.
> In absolute replacement, animals are not required at all at any stage. It
> follows ... that *absolute replacement may be regarded as the absolute ideal.*
> William Russell and Rex Burch (1959, p. 70: my italics)

## THE CONSTRUCTION OF A MODERN RESEARCH
## INSTITUTION

In previous chapters, I have emphasised the need for moral consideration
in all experiments which involve animals. Despite exhaustive attempts
by scientists, theologians, humane philosophers and others to define a
single ethical model for animal experimentation, none has proved comprehensive. This does not mean that such an ethic is not attainable – the
difficulty lies in individual perceptions of other animals, and to what
extent, if any, they ought to be included in our moral sphere. Albert
Schweitzer's 'reverence for life' and Peter Singer's 'animal interests' are
examples of ethics, derived in different ways, which have prepared the
ground for the erection of the modern research institution. Now, and into
the future, all such institutions will be staffed by scientists committed to
using animals (and sentient animals in particular) in experiments only
when it is absolutely necessary. The 'three Rs' of William Russell and Rex
Burch (1959) provide solid foundations for construction. Remember, it is
by introducing replacement alternatives at every opportunity, reducing
the numbers of animals involved in essential experiments and refining
procedures to minimise or eliminate suffering that scientists are best
able to justify their research.

## ABSOLUTE REPLACEMENT OR RELATIVE REPLACEMENT?

Estimating the total number of animals used in research, education
and safety testing each year is difficult. Not all countries report

comprehensive annual data or require institutions to engage in detailed statistical record keeping. Recent estimates of animals bred and/or used worldwide exceed 100 million per year (Knight 2008; Taylor *et al.* 2008; Akhtar 2015; Rossi 2015), but global estimates do not give sufficient detail about which species are used, or for what purpose. Without detailed information from all nations that use animals in experimentation, it is difficult to determine whether Russell and Burch's (1959) ideal of absolute replacement is coming into view.

However, the United Kingdom has kept detailed statistics on animal use for many years (see Chapter 2), and it is useful to explore its animal use trends. Currently, animal breeding for genetic alteration research, accounting for half of all experimental procedures completed each year (UK Home Office 2016), has resulted in an overall increase in animal use in the twenty-first century rather than a decrease. It is not known when such breeding for research will peak.

In the United Kingdom, 50 per cent of the animals involved in genetic alteration procedures are 'surplus' (UK Home Office 2016, pp. 9–10), and it is in this field of animal-based research that most reductions in the numbers of animals used can be made. Absolute replacement relies, therefore, on the development of radically new gene drive and gene alteration technologies that completely replace current methodologies where $F_1$ (and subsequent) generations need to be born. Could such discoveries perhaps lead to a halving of the total amount of scientific animal use in one go?

Will the interfaces between biology and engineering in fields such as synthetic biology and organ-on-a-chip technologies play a role here? Might novel *in silico* and biomimetic replacement alternatives or other converging technologies provide direction towards any goal of absolute replacement?

There are excellent reasons to continue to replace animals used in science with established alternatives; there are powerful reasons to actively seek next-generation alternatives. Some of these reasons are based in ethical discourse (Perry 2007; Ormandy, Dale and Griffin 2011; Gross and Tolba 2015) or a desire to improve welfare standards (Mellor 2015b, 2016); others also make good scientific sense (Hartung

2011; Davies 2012b). Seeking replacement alternatives must continue to be recognised as a core ethical principle underpinning modern animal experimentation. The search also represents the pro-science ideal that challenges scientists and bioengineers to create ethically superior experimental methods (Gauthier and Griffin 2005).

Was it naïve for Russell and Burch (1959) to posit that all animal experimentation may eventually cease? I don't believe so. While absolute replacement still remains an ideal, relative replacement continues apace. For example, in veterinary education, the use of computer simulations and supervised clinical placements that replace live animal experimentation and training is now widespread (Knight 2007; Lairmore and Ilkiw 2015). In the training of animal technicians, advanced skills in husbandry and enrichment are now the norm (Wolfensohn and Lloyd 2013); and research scientists are being actively encouraged to seek alternatives to animal models as a part of their education (Dewhurst 2008).

In safety testing, recent paradigm shifts away from *in vivo* testing have followed the regulatory changes designed to hasten the phase-out of cosmetic and other product testing using animals. The European Union now has far-reaching legislation banning cosmetic ingredients and products that have been newly tested using animals (EC Regulation No 1223/2009: Burden, Sewell and Chapman 2015). In 2014, India also banned the importation of cosmetic products and ingredients where animal testing had been part of their manufacturing process. In 2015, New Zealand passed the *Animal Welfare Amendment Act (No. 2)* which also includes a ban on domestic cosmetic product and ingredient testing using animals. Other countries, including Australia, are set to follow.

In 2007, the US National Research Council released a vision document for toxicological testing, *Toxicity Testing in the 21st Century: A Vision and a Strategy*. The emphasis in the USA is now on *in vitro* testing, computer modelling and a greatly reduced reliance on animal trials (Stephens and Mak 2014). The ethical principle of 'replacement' underpins this move. Whether it results only in 'relative replacement' or how long it takes to ultimately achieve 'absolute replacement' remains a challenge for current and future scientists.

CONCLUSIONS

This book has been written to help you to form your own opinions about many of the complex issues in animal experimentation. Some readers might be absolutist (wholly for or wholly against animal experiments); others will differ by degrees over the question of which animals ought to be used, and to what extent, for scientific purposes. Many may argue that non-human animals are used of necessity and that this practice ought to continue while suitable alternatives are sought.

In Chapter 2, Claude Bernard was quoted as asking why, in nineteenth-century society, when animals were used for food, transport, sport and entertainment, should they not also be used for scientific research. Contemporary use of animals has not changed greatly since then, so the question he posed in 1865 is as relevant today as it was then.

Most members of modern societies continue to condone (through their consumer purchases) intensive food animal production. This includes practices that present welfare challenges such as the confinement of pigs in sow stalls, and ethical challenges such as our societal acceptance of the killing of billions of unwanted day-old male chicks each year in the egg-laying industry[1]. We also continue to allow the use of animals for sport and entertainment at racetracks, rodeos and circuses where animals can be commodified. We do little in the form of public education campaigns to reduce the numbers of companion animals that are unwanted, abandoned and subsequently euthanised each year. As long as consumers in many countries continue to condone the exhaustive choices of shampoos, perfumes, cleaning products etc. we see on supermarket shelves, there will continue to be a need for high numbers of animals in safety testing. All of these uses of animals satisfy only present needs. Modern biomedicine offers potential solutions to future needs. It is built on a foundation of animal experimentation, and the public have consistently favoured its continuation.

Claude Bernard's assertion, of course, does not provide a justification for modern animal use that is beyond scrutiny. It can be argued that in

[1]Over 6.7 billion layer hens were used worldwide in 2013. A similar number of unwanted male chicks would have been born in the same year. www.wattagnet.com/Regional-trends-in-number-of-laying-hens-2000-13

our modern societies, reliance on non-human animals for food, entertainment, science and education is redundant. Indeed, many people are highlighting ethical and welfare issues associated with all such animal uses and questioning their continuation on the basis of inherent animal suffering. In science, education and industry, compromise solutions between the abolition of all experimentation and an uncontrolled use of research animals now emphasise the minimisation or elimination of suffering from essential experiments. Well-educated scientists now recognise that they have specific obligations to the research animals in their care and strive to ensure that the welfare of their subjects is a high priority.

I introduced this book with a quote by Miriam Rothschild. She recounted how the ethics of zoology were never an overt consideration for her educators in the mid-twentieth century. In the twenty-first century, the situation is changing drastically for the better. Research animals now are afforded more legislative protection, ethical consideration by scientists and scrutiny by the public than at any other time.

Increasingly, modern life science curricula are taking on board alternative teaching techniques. In some subjects, options are available for students who do not wish to participate in practical classes where experiments using animals are conducted. Animal welfare courses now form essential components of many veterinary training programmes. As the availability of alternatives to invasive procedures becomes more widespread in certain subjects (and that availability is advertised beforehand in course outlines), more students may fulfil their interests in life sciences without compromising their thoughtfully explored ethical stance.

However, students within such courses also must recognise their responsibilities. The education offered through the use of animals and animal tissues is not a right – it is a privilege given to them by an expectant society. It is important to recognise this and for students to conduct themselves appropriately in classes where animals are used. To this aim, the Australian and New Zealand Council for the Care of Animals in Research and Teaching has written a suite of ethical guidelines that I have reproduced at the end of this book (ANZCCART 2013). If you do not wish to participate in a practical class involving an animal experiment for ethical reasons, don't wait until you get to the class to voice your concerns. By then, an animal may already have been sourced or killed for you. See the subject teacher well ahead of time. Propose an alternative practical you would like to do instead of the scheduled dissection or live experiment. Show the staff your objections are rational and well-considered (see Knight 2011).

Some medical schools conduct special services to remember the people who have donated their bodies to science. Such services aim to instil in students humility and respect for the thoughtfulness of others. It would be nice to think the day will come when similar services are held for staff and students to mark the sacrifices made for our benefit by research animals. The humane consideration of the lives of other animals is honourable. Animal rights? Animal interests? Reverence for life? The terminology is unimportant: it is respect for other creatures that is of the utmost importance. Young scientists who carry this respect into their workplace will be instrumental in introducing future alternative methods which will continue the reform of animal experimentation to its ultimate conclusion – absolute replacement.

In the meantime, if you have chosen a career in a biological science, then you carry with you a responsibility to conduct yourselves and your research ethically. You have been given a trust by society in general which is not to be taken lightly. Remember, you have chosen an honourable profession – act honourably in all your dealings with research animals and do not lose sight of the sacrifice which we force them to make.

# Ethical guidelines for students in laboratory classes involving the use of animals or animal tissues

The following guidelines were produced by ANZCCART[1] with the recommendation that they be displayed prominently in student laboratories and included in laboratory manuals.

> The use of animals or animal tissues in laboratory classes is a privilege that brings with it responsibilities. These responsibilities go well beyond the need to avoid cruelty to animals and involve a genuine commitment to their welfare and a respect for the contribution they make to your learning. Outlined below are principles to consider in helping you to meet these responsibilities and to derive maximum benefit from the use of animals in laboratory classes.

## PRINCIPLES TO CONSIDER

### 1. Consider why animals or animal tissues are being used in the laboratory

The justification for using animals should be that their use is essential for the achievement of educational outcomes, while recognising the potential for harm to animals to achieve these outcomes. Consideration must be given to whether the educational outcomes could be achieved without the use of animals or animal tissues. Every student and staff member should be mindful of the 3Rs (Replacement, Reduction and Refinement) when working with animals.

### 2. Consider the requirements for animal welfare and animal handling

At all times the welfare of the animal you use is your responsibility, not just your teacher's responsibility. This can be considered as a 'duty of care'. If you are required to handle animals during a laboratory class, it

[1] www.adelaide.edu.au/ANZCCART/docs/aust-ethical-guide2013.pdf

is important to follow the instructions of staff in the correct handling and restraint techniques for the species with which you are working.

### 3. Consider the regulatory environment

The use of animals in research and teaching in Australia is regulated by State and Territory government legislation incorporating the *Australian code for the care and use of animals for scientific purposes*. The use of animals for research and teaching must first be approved by an Animal Ethics Committee (AEC). Gaining this approval involves justification for using animals (species and number), the means by which animals will be handled and, if required, humanely killed, and the potential research and educational outcomes of the work balanced against any potential harm to the animals used. The skills of the staff involved and the supervision of the students are also evaluated. In fact, the questions raised by AECs should be those asked by each student regarding the use of animals for their education.

### 4. Consider your own views in using animals or animal tissues in the laboratory

You should discuss the use of animals or animal tissues with other students and staff. Opinions should be formed and aired, with appropriate justification, in an open and accepting environment. You should feel free to make suggestions that might improve future laboratory classes, and to this end, student opinion regarding the use of animals in teaching should be encouraged.

### 5. Consider your responsibility to make sure that good use is made of the learning opportunity

You should know what underlying principles are being taught in the class and understand the details that illustrate those principles. This involves reading background material from lecture notes, references and laboratory manuals before coming to class and being generally prepared to maximise the learning experience. Use every opportunity, within the approved scope of the class, to develop manual, observational and recording skills.

# References

Abraham, M.H., Hassanisadi, M., Jalali-Heravi, M., Ghafourian, T., Cain, W.S. and Cometto-Muniz, J.E. 2003. Draize rabbit eye test compatibility with eye irritation thresholds in humans: a quantitative structure-activity relationship analysis. *Toxicological Sciences* **76**: 384–391.

Adams, R. 1977. *The Plague Dogs*. Harmondsworth: Penguin.

Akhtar, A. 2015. The flaws and human harms of animal experimentation. *Cambridge Quarterly of Healthcare Ethics* **24**: 407–419.

American Medical Association Council on Scientific Affairs 1989. Council report on animals in research. *Journal of the American Medical Association* **261**: 3602–3606.

Animal Welfare Committee 2007. *National Health and Medical Research Council Guidelines for the Generation, Breeding, Care, and Use of Genetically Modified and Cloned Animals for Scientific Purposes*. Canberra: Australian Government.

Anon. 1992. Scientific procedures on living animals, cited in Porter, D.G. Ethical scores for animal experiments. *Nature* **356**: 101–102.

Ashall, V. and Millar, K. 2014. Endpoint matrix: a conceptual tool to promote consideration of the multiple dimensions of humane endpoints. *Alternatives to Animal Experimentation* **31**: 209–213.

Association for the Study of Animal Behaviour 2012. Guidelines for the treatment of animals in behavioural research and teaching. *Animal Behaviour* **83**: 301–309.

Australian and New Zealand Council for the Care of Animals in Research and Teaching 2013. Ethical guidelines for students in laboratory classes using animals or animal tissues. www.adelaide.edu.au/ANZCCART/docs/aust-ethical-guide2013.pdf.

Australian Government, Senate Select Committee on Animal Welfare 1989. *Animal Experimentation*. Canberra: Australian Government Publishing Service.

Bacon, F. 1605/2001. *The Advancement of Learning (1605)*, Gould S.J. (ed.). New York: Random House.

Bailey, K.R., Rustay, N.R. and Crawley, J.N. 2006. Behavioral phenotyping of transgenic and knockout mice: practical concerns and potential pitfalls. *ILAR Journal* **47**: 124–131.

Baker, K.C. and Dettmer, A.M. 2016. The well-being of laboratory non-human primates. *American Journal of Primatology* doi:10.1002/ajp.22520.

Balcombe, J.P., Barnard, N.D. and Sandusky, C. 2004. Laboratory routines cause animal stress. *Journal of the American Association for Laboratory Animal Science* **43**: 42–51.

Balls, M. 1990. Recent progress toward reducing the use of animal experimentation in biomedical research. In Garattini, S. and van Bekkum, D.W. (eds.), *The Importance of Animal Experimentation for Safety and Biomedical Research*, pp. 223–235. Dordrecht: Kluwer.

Battye, J. 1994. Ethics and animal welfare - where do we go from here? In Baker, R.M., Mellor, D.J. and Nicol, A.M. (eds.) *Animal Welfare in the Twenty-First Century: Ethical, Educational and Scientific Challenges*, pp. 3–10. Adelaide: ANZCCART.

Baumans, V., Coke, C., Green, J., Moreau, E., Morton, D., Patterson-Kane, E., Reinhardt, A., Reinhardt, V. and Van Loo, P. (eds.) 2007. *Making Lives Easier for Animals in Research Labs*. Washington DC: Animal Welfare Institute. www.awionline.org/pubs/LAREF/LAREF-bk.html

Bayne, K. and Würbel, H. 2014. The impact of environmental enrichment on the outcome variability and scientific validity of laboratory animal studies. *Scientific and Technical Review of the Office International des Epizooties (Paris)* **33**: 273–280.

Bayne, K., Ramachandra, G.S., Rivera, E.A. and Wang, J. 2015. The evolution of animal welfare and the 3Rs in Brazil, China, and India. *Journal of the American Association for Laboratory Animal Science* **54**: 181–191.

Behrens, K.G. 2014. Genetic modification (GMOs): Animals. In ten Have, H. (ed.) *Encyclopedia of Global Bioethics*, pp. 1–10. doi:10.1007/978-3-319-05544-2_209-1.

Bekoff, M. (ed.) 2013. *Ignoring Nature No More: The Case for Compassionate Conservation*. Chicago: University of Chicago Press.

Benassi, L., Bertazzoni, G. and Seidenari, S. 1999. *In vitro* testing of tensides employing monolayer cultures: a comparison with results of patch tests on human volunteers. *Contact Dermatitis* **40**: 38–44.

Benison, S. 1970. In defense of medical research. *Harvard Medical, Alumni Bulletin* **44**: 16–23.

Bentham, J. 1789/1970. An introduction to the principles of morals and legislation. In Burns, J.H. and Hart, H.L.A. (eds.), *The Collected Works of Jeremy Bentham*, Vol. 2.1. London: Athlone.

Bernard, C. 1865/1957. *An Introduction to the Study of Experimental Medicine*, trans. Greene, H.C., 1957. New York: Dover.

Bilbo, S.D. and Nelson, R.J. 2001. Behavioral phenotyping of transgenic and knockout animals: a cautionary tale. *Lab Animal* **30**: 24–29.

Birch, C. 1993. *Regaining Compassion for Humanity and Nature*. Kensington: New South Wales University Press, pp. 86–96.

Bliss, M. 1982. *The Discovery of Insulin*. Chicago: University of Chicago Press.

Brabazon, J. 1976. *Albert Schweitzer: A Biography*. London: Victor Gollancz.

Britt, D. 1984. Ethics, ethical committees and animal experimentation. *Nature* **311**: 503–506.

Bronowski, J. 1956. *Science and Human Values*, revised edition 1965. New York: Harper and Row.

Brown, M.J. and Murray, K.A. 2006. Phenotyping of genetically engineered mice: humane, ethical, environmental, and husbandry issues. *ILAR Journal* **47**: 118–123.

Bruce, D. and Bruce, A. 2003. Genetic engineering and animal welfare. In Armstrong, S.J. and Botzler, R.G. (eds.), *The Animal Ethics Reader*, pp. 313–322. London: Routledge.

Buehr, M., Hjorth, J.P. and Hansen, A.K. 2003. Genetically modified laboratory animals – what welfare problems do they face? *Journal of Applied Animal Welfare Science* **6**: 319–338.

Burden, N., Sewell, F. and Chapman, K. 2015. Testing chemical safety: what is needed to ensure the widespread application of non-animal approaches? *PLOS Biology* **13**(5) e1002156. doi:10.1371/journal.pbio.1002156.

Calisi, R.M. and Bentley, G.E. 2009. Lab and field experiments: are they the same animal? *Hormones and Behavior* **56**: 1–10.

Callicott, J.B. 1989. *In Defense of the Land Ethic: Essays in Environmental Philosophy*. New York: State University of New York Press.

Caplan, A. 1989. Cited in *Animal Experimentation, Australian Government, Senate Select Committee on Animal Welfare*. Canberra: Australian Government Publishing Service.

**CIOMS and ICLAS**, Council for International Organizations of Medical Sciences (CIOMS), International Council for Laboratory Animal Science (ICLAS) 2012. *International Guiding Principles for Biomedical Research Involving Animals*. www.cioms.ch.

**Clark, S.R.L.** 1984. *The Moral Status of Animals*. Oxford: Oxford University Press.

**Clark, S.R.L.** 1997. *Animals and Their Moral Standing*. London: Routledge.

**Cloutier, S., Panksepp, J. and Newberry, R.C.** 2012. Playful handling by caretakers reduces fear of humans in the laboratory rat. *Applied Animal Behaviour Science* **140**: 161–171.

**Cordelli, E., Fresegna, A.M., D'Alessio, A., Spano, M., Villani, P. and Pacchierotti, F.** 2007. A new *in vitro* method to assess DNA damage in sperm as an alternative to animal testing in reproductive toxicology. *Toxicology Letters* **172**: S76. doi:10.1016/j.toxlet.2007.05.218.

**Cottingham, J.** 1978. A brute to the brutes?: Descartes' treatment of animals. *Philosophy* **53**: 551–559.

**Cranefield, P.F.** 1974. *The Way In and the Way Out: François Magendie, Charles Bell, and the Roots of the Spinal Nerves*. New York: Futura.

**Cressey, D.** 2011. Animal research: battle scars. *Nature* **470**: 452–453.

**Crettaz von Roten, F.** 2012. Public perceptions of animal experimentation across Europe. *Public Understanding of Science* **22**: 691–703.

**Curtright, A., Rosser, M., Goh, S. Keown, B., Wagner, E., Sharifi, J., Raible, D.W. and Dhaka, A.** 2015. Modeling nociception in zebrafish: a way forward for unbiased analgesic discovery. *PloS One* **10**(1): e0116766. doi:10.1371/journal.pone.0116766.

**Daneshian, M., Busquet, F., Hartung, T. and Leist, M.** 2015. Animal use for science in Europe. *Alternatives to Animal Experimentation* **32**: 261–274.

**Darwin, C.** 1859/2009. *On the Origin of Species by Natural Selection*. New York: Oxford University Press.

**Darwin, C.** 1871/2004. *The Descent of Man, and Selection in Relation to Sex*. London: Penguin Classics.

**Darwin, C.** 1881/1985. *The Formation of Vegetable Mould, through the Action of Worms*. Facsimile of the first edition reprinted by the University of Chicago Press, Chicago.

**Daston, G., Knight, D.J., Schwarz, M., Gocht, T., Thomas, R.S., Mahony, C. and Whelan, M.** 2015. SEURAT: Safety evaluation ultimately replacing animal testing – recommendations for future research in the field of predictive toxicology. *Archives of Toxicology* **89**: 15–23.

**Davies, J.** (ed.) 2012a. *Replacing Animal Models: A Practical Guide to Creating and Using Culture-based Biomimetic Alternatives*. Hoboken, NJ: John Wiley.

**Davies, J.** 2012b. Potential advantages of using biomimetic alternatives. In Davies, J. (ed.) *Replacing Animal Models: A Practical Guide to Creating and Using Culture-based Biomimetic Alternatives*, pp. 3–11. Hoboken, NJ: John Wiley.

**Denton, D.** 1993. *The Pinnacle of Life: Consciousness and Self-Awareness in Humans and Animals*. Sydney: Allen and Unwin.

**Descartes, R.** 1637/1984. *Discours de la Méthode*, trans. Curtis, D. London: Grant and Cutler.

**Dewhurst, D.** 2008. Is it possible to meet the learning objectives of undergraduate pharmacology classes with non-animal models? *Alternatives to Animal Testing and Experimentation* **14**: 207–212.

**Di Marco, P.N., Howell, J.McC. and Dorling, P.R.** 1984. Bovine glycogenosis type II. Biochemical and morphological characteristics of skeletal muscle in culture. *Neuropathology and Applied Neurobiology* **10**: 379–395.

**Draize, J.H., Woodward, G. and Calvery, H.O.** 1944. Methods for the study of irritation and toxicity of substances applied topically to the skin and mucous membranes. *Journal of Pharmacology and Experimental Therapy* **82**: 377–390.

Duckworth, W.L.H., Lyons, M.C. and Towers, B. (eds.) 1962. *Galen, On Anatomical Procedures: The Later Books*. Cambridge: Cambridge University Press.

Eisemann, C.H., Jorgensen, W.K., Merritt, D.J., Rice, M.J., Cribb, B.W., Webb, P.D. and Zalucki, M.P. 1984. Do insects feel pain? - A biological view. *Experientia* **40**: 164–167.

Elwood, R.W. 2011. Pain and suffering in invertebrates? *ILAR Journal* **52**: 175–184.

Enders, J.F., Weller, T.H. and Robbins, F.C. 1949. Cultivation of the Lansing strain of poliomyelitis virus in cultures of various human embryonic tissue. *Science* **109**: 85–87.

European Commission 2009. EC Regulation No 1223/2009 of the European Parliament and of the Council of 30 November 2009 on cosmetic products. In *Official Journal of the European Union*. Brussels: EC, 2009, pp. 52–59.

European Commission 2010. Directive 2010/63/EU of the European Parliament and of the Council of 22 September 2010 on the protection of animals used for scientific purposes. In *Official Journal of the European Union*. Brussels: EC, 2010, pp. 33–79.

European Commission 2013. *Animals Used for Scientific Purposes*. Seventh report on the statistics on the number of animals used for experimental and other scientific purposes in the member states of the European Union. http://ec.europa.eu/environment/chemicals/lab_animals/reports_en.htm.

Feng, W., Dai, Y., Mou, L., Cooper, D.K.C., Shi, D. and Cai, Z. 2015. The potential of the combination of CRISPR/Cas9 and pluripotent stem cells to provide human organs from chimaeric pigs. *International Journal of Molecular Science* **16**: 6545–6556.

Fisher, J.A. 1987. Taking sympathy seriously: a defense of our moral psychology toward animals. *Environmental Ethics* **9**: 197–215.

Fleetwood, G., Chlebus, M., Coenen, J., Dudoignon, N., Lecerf, C., Maisonneuve, C. and Robinson, S. 2015. Making progress and gaining momentum in global 3Rs efforts: how the European pharmaceutical industry is contributing. *Journal of the American Association for Laboratory Animal Science* **54**: 192–197.

Flemming, A.H. 1984. *Ethical Considerations*, cited in US Congress, Office of Technology Assessment, 1986, *Alternatives to Animal Use in Research, Testing, and Education*, p. 74. New York: Marcel Dekker.

Flexner, S. and Lewis, P.A. 1909. The transmission of acute poliomyelitis to monkeys. *Journal of the American Medical Association* **53**(20): 1639. doi:10.1001/jama.1909.92550200027002g.

FRAME Toxicity Committee 1991. Animals and alternatives in toxicology: present status and future prospects. *Alternatives to Laboratory Animals* **19**: 116–138.

Franco, N.H. 2013. Animal experiments in biomedical research: a historical perspective. *Animals* **3**: 238–273.

Franco, N.H. and Olsson, I.A.S. 2014. Scientists and the 3Rs: attitudes to animal use in biomedical research and the effect of mandatory training in laboratory animal science. *Laboratory Animals* **48**: 50–60.

Franco N.H., Correia-Neves M. and Olsson I.A.S. 2012. How "humane" is your endpoint?—Refining the science-driven approach for termination of animal studies of chronic infection. *PLoS Pathogens* **8**(1): e1002399. doi:10.1371/journal.ppat.1002399.

Franklin, A. 2007. Human-nonhuman animal relationships in Australia: an overview of results from the first national survey and follow-up case studies 2000–2004. *Society and Animals* **15**: 7–27.

French, R.D. 1975. *Antivivisection and Medical Science in Victorian Society*. Princeton, NJ: Princeton University Press.

French, R.D. 1978. Animal experimentation: historical aspects. In Reich, W.T. (ed.), *Encyclopedia of Bioethics*, Vol. 1, pp. 75–79. New York: Free Press.

French, R.D. 1999. *Dissection and Vivisection in the European Renaissance*. Aldershot, UK: Ashgate Publishing.

Galen, 1956. *On Anatomical Procedures*, trans. Singer, C. Oxford: Oxford University Press.

Galvin, S.L. and Herzog, H.A. 1998. Attitudes and dispositional optimism of animal rights demonstrators. *Society and Animals* 6: 1–11.

Gärtner, K., Büttner, D., Döhler, K., Friedel, R., Lindena, J. and Trautschold, I. 1980. Stress response of rats to handling and experimental procedures. *Laboratory Animals* 14: 267–274.

Gaughen, S. (ed.) 2005. *Animal Rights: Contemporary Issues Companion*. Farmington Hills, MI: Greenhaven Press.

Gauthier, C. and Griffin, G. 2005. Using animals in research, testing and teaching. *Scientific and Technical Review of the Office International des Epizooties* 24: 735–745.

Gerner, I., Liebsch, M. and Spielmann, H. 2005. Assessment of the eye irritating properties of chemicals by applying alternatives to the Draize rabbit eye test: the use of QSARs and *in vitro* tests for the classification of eye irritation. *Alternatives to Laboratory Animals* 33: 215–237.

Goodman, J.R. and Sanders, C.R. 2011. In favor of tipping the balance: animal rights activists in defense of residential picketing. *Society and Animals* 19: 137–155.

Gott, M. and Monamy, V. 2004. Ethics and transgenesis: towards a policy framework incorporating intrinsic objections and societal perceptions. *Alternative to Laboratory Animals* 32, Supplement 1A: 391–396.

Graham, D.M. 2016. Methods for measuring pain in laboratory animals. *Lab Animal* 45: 99–101.

Grant, L., Hopkinson, P., Jennings, G. and Jenner, F.A. 1971. Period of adjustment of rats used for experimental studies. *Nature* 232: 135.

Gray, G.E., Laher, F., Lazarus, E., Ensoli, B. and Corey, L. 2016. Approaches to preventative and therapeutic HIV vaccines. *Current Opinion in Virology* 17: 104–109.

Gross, D. and Tolba, R.H. 2015. Ethics in animal-based research. *European Surgical Research* 55: 43–57.

Gruen, L. 1991. Animals. In Singer, P. (ed.), *A Companion to Ethics*, pp. 343–353. Oxford: Blackwell Reference.

Gruen, L. 2011. *Ethics and Animals: An Introduction*. New York: Cambridge University Press.

Gruen, L. 2014. *The Moral Status of Animals, The Stanford Encyclopedia of Philosophy* (Fall 2014 Edition), Zlatan, E.N. (ed.). http://plato.stanford.edu/archives/fall2014/entries/moral-animal/.

Guillén, J., Prins, J.B., Smith, D. and Degryse, A.D. 2014. The European framework on research animal welfare regulations and guidelines. In Guillén, J. (ed.), *Laboratory Animals: Regulations and Recommendations for Global Collaborative Research*, pp. 117–188. New York: Elsevier.

Hakkinen, P.J. and Green, D.K. 2002. Alternatives to animal testing: information resources via the internet and world wide web. *Toxicology* 173: 3–11.

Harmon, T.M., Fisher, K.A., McGlynn, M.G., Stover, J., Warren, M.J., Teng, Y. and Näveke, A. 2016. Exploring the potential health impact and cost-effectiveness of AIDS vaccine within a comprehensive HIV/AIDS response in low- and middle-income countries. *PLoS ONE* 11(1): e0146387. doi:10.1371/journal.pone.0146387.

Hartung, T. 2011. From alternative methods to a new toxicology. *European Journal of Pharmaceutics and Biopharmaceutics* 77: 338–349.

Harvey, W. 1628/1978. *Exercitatio anatomica de motu cordis et sanguinis in animalibus:* being a facsimile of the 1628 Francofurti edition, together with the Keynes English translation of 1928. Birmingham, AL: Classics of Medicine Library.

Hodgson, J.C. and Koh, L.P. 2016. Best practice for minimising unmanned aerial vehicle disturbance to wildlife in biological field research. *Current Biology* **26**: R404-R405 doi:10.1016/j.cub.2016.04.001.

Hoggatt, J., Hoggatt, A.F., Tate, T.A., Fortman, J. and Pelus, L.M. 2016. Bleeding the laboratory mouse: not all methods are equal. *Experimental Hematology* **44**: 132–137.

Hooijmans, C.R., Tillema, A., Leenaars, M. and Ritskes-Hoitinga, M. 2010. Enhancing search efficiency by means of a search filter for finding all studies on animal experimentation in PubMed. *Laboratory Animals* **44**: 170–175.

Howell, J.McC., Dorling, P.R. and Cook, R.D. 1983. Generalized glycogenosis type II. *Comparative Pathology Bulletin* **15**: 2–4.

Hubrecht, R.C. 2014. *The Welfare of Animals Used in Research: Practice and Ethics*. Oxford: Wiley-Blackwell.

Hubrecht, R.C. and Kirkwood, J. (eds.) 2010. *The UFAW Handbook on the Care and Management of Laboratory and Other Research Animals*, eighth edition. Hoboken, NJ: Wiley-Blackwell.

Hume, C.W. 1962. *Man and Beast*. London: Universities Federation for Animal Welfare.

Humphrey, N.K. 1983. *Consciousness Regained: Chapters in the Development of Mind*. Oxford: Oxford University Press.

Infield, L. 1963. *Immanuel Kant: Lectures on Ethics*. New York: Harper and Row.

Jackson, S.J., Andrews, N., Ball, D., Bellantuono, I., Gray, J., Hachoumi, L., Holmes, A., Latcham, J., Petrie, A., Potter, P., Rice, A., Ritchie, A., Stewart, M., Strepka, C., Yeoman, M. and Chapman, K. 2016. Does age matter? The impact of rodent age on study outcomes. *Laboratory Animals* doi:10.1177/0023677216653984.

Joffe, A.R., Bara, M., Anton, N. and Nobis, N. 2016. The ethics of animal research: a survey of the public and scientists in North America. *BMC Medical Ethics* **17**: 17 doi:10.1186/s12910-016-0100-x.

Jung, K., Lee, S., Jang, W., Jung, H., Heo, Y., Park, Y., Bae, S., Lim, K. and Seok, S. 2014. KeraSkin$^{TM}$-VM: a novel reconstructed human epidermis model for skin irritation tests. *Toxicology in Vitro* **28**: 742–750.

Kar, S. and Roy, K. 2014. Quantification of contributions of molecular fragments for eye irritation of organic chemicals using QSAR study. *Computers in Biology and Medicine* **48**: 102–108.

Kew, O. 2012. Reaching the last one per cent: progress and challenges in global polio eradication. *Current Opinion in Virology* **2**: 188–198.

Kilkenny, C., Browne, W.J., Cuthill, I.C., Emerson, M. and Altman, D.G. 2010. Improving bioscience research reporting: the ARRIVE guidelines for reporting animal research. *PloS Biology* **8**(6): e1000412. doi:10.1371/journal.pbio.1000412.

Kilkenny, C., Parsons, N., Kadyszewski, E., Festing, M.F.W., Cuthill, I.C., Fry, D., Hutton, J. and Altman, D.G. 2009. Survey of the quality of experimental design, statistical analysis and reporting of research using animals. *PloS One* **4**(11): e7824. doi:10.1371/journal.pone.0007824.

Kitchell, R.L. and Erickson, H.H. 1983. Introduction. In Kitchell, R.L. and Erickson, H.H. (eds.), *Animal Pain: Perception and Alleviation*, p. vii. Bethesda: American Physiological Society.

Knight, A. 2007. The effectiveness of humane teaching methods in veterinary education. *Alternatives to Animal Testing and Experimentation* **24**: 91–109.

Knight, A. 2008. 127 million non-human vertebrates used worldwide for scientific purposes in 2005. *Alternatives to Laboratory Animals* **36**: 494–496.

Knight, A. 2011. *The Costs and Benefits of Animal Experiments*. Basingstoke, UK: Palgrave MacMillan.

Lairmore, M.D. and Ilkiw, J. 2015. Animals used in research and education, 1966–2016: evolving attitudes, policies, and relationships. *Journal of Veterinary Medical Education* 42: 425–440.

Langley, G. 1989. Plea for a sensitive science. In Langley, G. (ed.), *Animal Experimentation: The Consensus Changes*, pp. 193–218. Oxford: MacMillan Press.

Lappin, G., Noveck, R. and Burt, T. 2013. Microdosing and drug development: past, present and future. *Expert Opinion on Drug Metabolism and Toxicology* 9: 817–834.

Leahman, J., Latter, J. and Clemence, M. 2014. *Attitudes to Animal Research in 2014: A Report by Ipsos MORI for the Department for Business Innovation and Skills*. London: Ipsos MORI, Social Research Institute.

Lederer, S.E. 1987. The controversy over animal experimentation in America, 1880–1914. In Rupke, N.A. (ed.), *Vivisection in Historical Perspective*, pp. 236–258. London: Croom Helm.

Leopold, A. 1949. *A Sand County Almanac*. Oxford: Oxford University Press.

Lindsjö, J., Fahlman, A. and Törnqvist, E. 2016. Animal welfare from mouse to moose – implementing the principles of the 3Rs in wildlife research. *Journal of Wildlife Diseases* 52(2) Suppl.: S65-S77 doi:10.7589/52.2S.S65.

Linzey, A. 1989. Reverence, responsibility and rights. In Paterson, D. and Palmer M. (eds.), *The Status of Animals: Ethics, Education and Welfare*, pp. 20–50. Oxford: CABI.

Linzey, A. and Clarke, P.A.B. 2004. *Animal Rights: A Historical Anthology*. Irvington, NY: Columbia University Press.

Littin, K.E. 2010. Animal welfare and pest control: meeting both conservation and animal welfare goals. *Animal Welfare* 19: 171–176.

Maehle, A-H. and Tröhler, U. 1987. Animal experimentation from antiquity to the end of the eighteenth century: attitudes and arguments. In Rupke, N.A. (ed.), *Vivisection in Historical Perspective*, pp. 14–47. London: Croom-Helm.

Manning, H. 1887/1934. *Cardinal Manning, Archbishop of Westminster on Vivisection*. London: Victoria Street Society for the Protection of Animals from Vivisection. Republished Melbourne.

Mather, J.A. 2011. Philosophical background of attitudes toward and treatment of invertebrates. *ILAR Journal* 52: 205–212.

Medina, L.V., Coenen, J. and Kastello, M.D. 2015. Global 3Rs efforts – making progress and gaining momentum. *Journal of the American Association for Laboratory Animal Science* 54: 115–118.

Mellor, D.J. 2015a. Positive animal welfare states and encouraging environment-focused and animal-to-animal interactive behaviours. *New Zealand Veterinary Journal* 63: 9–16.

Mellor, D.J. 2015b. Positive animal welfare states and reference standards for welfare assessment. *New Zealand Veterinary Journal* 63: 17–23.

Mellor, D.J. 2016. Updating animal welfare thinking: moving beyond the "five freedoms" towards "a life worth living." *Animals* 6: 21. doi:10.3390/ani6030021.

Mellor, D., Patterson-Kane, K. and Stafford, K.J. 2009. *The Sciences of Animal Welfare*. Oxford: Wiley-Blackwell.

Miles, A., Berthet, A., Hopf, N.B., Gilliet, M., Raffoul, W., Vernez, D. and Spring, P. 2014. A new alternative method for testing skin irritation using a human skin model: a pilot study. *Toxicology in Vitro* 28: 240–247.

Mitchell, A. 2001. How to measure welfare of transgenic farm animals. Proceedings of a workshop, *The Welfare of Transgenic Animals*, p. 20. Adelaide: ANZCCART.

**Moberg, G.P.** 2000. Biological response to stress: implications for animal welfare. In Moberg, G.P. and Mench, J.A. (eds.), *The Biology of Animal Stress: Basic Principles and Implications for Animal Welfare*, pp. 1–22. Wallingford, UK: CAB International.

**Monamy, V.** 2007. Hot iron branding of seals and sea lions: why the ban will remain. *Australian Veterinary Journal* **85**: 485–486.

**Monamy, V. and Gott, M.** 2001. Practical and ethical considerations for students conducting ecological research involving wildlife. *Austral Ecology* **26**: 293–300.

**Morton, D.B.** 2000. A systematic approach for establishing humane endpoints. *ILAR Journal* **41**: 80–86.

**Morton, D.B. and Griffiths, P.H.M.** 1985. Guidelines on the recognition of pain, distress and discomfort in experimental animals and an hypothesis for assessment. *Veterinary Record* **116**: 431–436.

**Mukerjee, M.** 1997. Trends in animal research. *Scientific American* **276**: 86–93.

**Nash, R.F.** 1990. *The Rights of Nature*. Sydney: Primavera Press.

**National Animal Ethics Advisory Committee (NAEAC)** 2012. *Guide to the Preparation of Codes of Ethical Conduct*. www.mpi.govt.nz/protection-and-response/animal-welfare/animals-in-research-testing-teaching/.

**National Centre for the Replacement Refinement and Reduction of Animals in Research** 2006. *NC3Rs Guidelines: Non-Human Primate Accommodation, Care and Use*. London: National Centre for the Replacement, Refinement and Reduction of Animals in Research. www.nc3rs.org.uk/non-human-primate-accommodation-care-and-use.

**National Health and Medical Research Council** 1990. *Strategies for Minimising the Numbers of Animals used in Research Projects*. Canberra: Australian Government Printer.

**National Health and Medical Research Council** 2013. *Australian Code for the Care and Use of Animals for Scientific Purposes*, eighth edition. Canberra: National Health and Medical Research Council.

**National Institutes of Health** 2005. *Enrichment for Non-Human Primates*. Washington DC: Office of Laboratory Animal Welfare. http://grants.nih.gov/grants/olaw/Enrichment_for_Nonhuman_Primates.pdf.

**National Institutes of Health** 2015. *Public Health Service Policy on Humane Care and Use of Laboratory Animals*. Bethesda, Maryland: U.S. Department of Health and Human Services. http://grants.nih.gov/grants/olaw/references/phspolicylabanimals.pdf.

**National Research Council** 1985. *Models for Biomedical Research: A New Perspective*. Washington DC: National Academy Press.

**National Research Council** 1988. *Use of Laboratory Animals in Biomedical and Behavioral Research*. Washington DC: National Academy Press.

**National Research Council** 2007. *Toxicity Testing in the 21$^{st}$ Century: A Vision and a Strategy*. Washington DC: National Academies Press.

**National Research Council** 2008. *Recognition and Alleviation of Distress in Laboratory Animals*. Washington DC: National Academies Press.

**National Research Council** 2011. *Guide for the Care and Use of Laboratory Animals*, eighth edition, Washington DC: National Academies Press.

**Nuffield Council on Bioethics** 2016. *Genome Editing: An Ethical Review*. London: Nuffield Council on Bioethics.

**OECD** 2012. *Fish Toxicity Testing Framework*. OECD Series on Testing and Assessment, No. 171 ENV/JM/MONO(2012)16. Paris: Organisation for Economic Cooperation and Development.

**Orlans, F.B.** 1993. *In the Name of Science: Issues in Responsible Animal Experimentation*. New York: Oxford University Press.

Ormandy, E.H. and Schuppli, C.A. 2014. Public attitudes toward animal research: a review. *Animals* 4: 391–408.

Ormandy, E.H., Dale, J. and Griffin, G. 2011. Genetic engineering of animals: ethical issues, including welfare concerns. *Canadian Veterinary Journal* 52: 544–550.

Ormandy, E.H., Schuppli, C.A. and Weary, D.M. 2012. Factors affecting people's acceptance of the use of zebrafish and mice in research. *Alternatives to Laboratory Animals* 40: 321–333.

Osterrieder, S.K., Kent, C.S., Anderson, C.J.R., Parnum, I.M. and Robinson, R.W. 2015. Whisker spot patterns: a noninvasive method of individual identification of Australian sea lions (*Neophoca cinerea*). *Journal of Mammalogy* 96: 988–997.

Parker, R.M.A. and Browne, W.J. 2014. The place of experimental design and statistics in the 3Rs. *ILAR Journal* 55: 477–485.

Paton, W.D.M. 1993. *Man and Mouse: Animals in Medical Research*, second edition. Oxford: Oxford University Press.

Paul, E., Sikes, R.S., Beaupre, S.J. and Wingfield, J.C. 2015. Animal welfare policy: implementation in the context of wildlife research – policy review and discussion of fundamental issues. *ILAR Journal* 56: 312–334.

Perry, P. 2007. The ethics of animal research: a UK perspective. *ILAR Journal* 48: 42–46.

Phillips, M.T. and Sechzer, J.A. 1989. *Animal Research and Ethical Conflict: An Analysis of the Scientific Literature 1966–1986*. New York: Springer-Verlag.

Pifer, L., Shimizu, K. and Pifer, R. 1994. Public attitudes toward animal research: some international comparisons. *Society and Animals* 2: 95–113.

Plint, A.C., Moher, D., Morrison, A., Schulz, K., Altman, D.G., Hill, C. and Gaboury, I. 2006. Does the CONSORT checklist improve the quality of reports of randomised controlled trials? A systematic review. *Medical Journal of Australia* 185: 263–267.

Poling, A., Schlinger, H., Starin, S. and Blakely, E. 1990. *Psychology: A Behavioral Overview*. New York: Plenum Press.

Porter, D.G. 1992. Ethical scores for animal experiments. *Nature* 356: 101–102.

Poumay, Y. and Coquette, A. 2007. Modelling the human epidermis *in vitro*: tools for basic and applied research. *Archives of Dermatological Research* 298: 361–369.

Regan, T. 1981. Animal rights and animal experimentation. In Basson, M.D. (ed.), *Rights and Responsibilities in Modern Medicine*, pp. 69–83. New York: Alan R. Liss.

Regan, T. 1982. *All That Dwell Therein: Animal Rights and Environmental Ethics*. Berkeley: University of California Press.

Regan, T. 1983. *The Case for Animal Rights*. Berkeley: University of California Press.

Regan, T. 1985. The case for animal rights. In Singer, P. (ed.), *In Defense of Animals*, pp. 13–26. Oxford: Basil Blackwell.

Regan, T. 1990. The struggle for animal rights. In Clarke, P.A.B. and Linzey, A. (eds.), *Political Theory and Animal Rights*, pp. 176–186. London: Pluto Press.

Regan, T. and Singer, P. (eds.) 1976. *Animal Rights and Human Obligations*. Englewood Cliffs, NJ: Prentice-Hall.

Remfry, J. 1987. Ethical aspects of animal experimentation. In Tuffery, A.A. (ed.), *Laboratory Animals: An Introduction for New Experimenters*, pp. 5–19. Chichester: John Wiley and Sons.

Riordan, S.M., Heruth, D.P., Zhang, L.Q. and Ye, S.Q. 2015. Application of CRISPR/Cas9 for biomedical discoveries. *Cell & Bioscience* 5: 33. doi:10.1186/s13578-015-0027-9.

Rodd, R. 1990. *Biology, Ethics and Animals*. Oxford: Clarendon Press.

Rollin, B.E. 1981. *Animal Rights and Human Morality*. New York: Prometheus.

Rolston, H. 1988. *Environmental Ethics: Duties to and Values in the Natural World*. Philadelphia: Temple University Press.

Rose, M. and Adams, D. 1989. Evidence for pain and suffering in other animals. In G. Langley (ed.), *Animal Experimentation: The Consensus Changes*, pp. 42–71. Oxford: MacMillan Press.

Rosenfield, L.C. 1940. *From Beast-Machine to Man-Machine*. Oxford: Oxford University Press.

Rossi, J. 2015. Research: animals. *Encyclopedia of Global Bioethics* doi:10.1007/978-3-319-05544-2_373-1.

Rothschild, M. 1986. *Animals and Man. The Romanes Lecture for 1984–85*. Oxford: Clarendon Press.

Rowan, A.N. 1984. *Of Mice, Models and Men: A Critical Evaluation of Animal Research*. Albany, NY: State University of New York Press.

Rowan, A.N. and Rollin, B.E. 1983. Animal research - for and against: a philosophical, social, and historical perspective. *Perspectives in Biology and Medicine* 27: 1–17.

RSPCA and LASA 2015. *Guiding Principles on Good Practice for Animal Welfare and Ethical Review Bodies*. A report by the RSPCA Research Animals Department and LASA Education, Training and Ethics Section. (M. Jennings, ed.).

Rubin, S.A. 2011. Toward replacement of the monkey neurovirulence test in vaccine safety testing. *Procedia in Vaccinology* 5: 261–265.

Rupke, N.A. 1987. Introduction. In Rupke, N.A. (ed.), *Vivisection in Historical Perspective*, pp. 1–13. London: Croom-Helm.

Russell, W.M.S. and Burch, R.L. 1959/1992. *The Principles of Humane Experimental Technique*. London: UFAW.

Rutherford, K.M.D. 2002. Assessing pain in animals. *Animal Welfare* 11: 31–53.

Ryder, R.D. 1975. *Victims of Science: The Use of Animals in Research*. London: Davis-Poynter.

Ryder, R.D. 2000. *Animal Revolution: Changing Attitudes towards Speciesism*, second edition. Oxford: Berg Publishers.

Sagan, C. and Druyan, A. 1992. *Shadows of Forgotten Ancestors: A Search for Who We Are*. Sydney: Random House.

Schweitzer, A. 1936. *Indian Thought and Its Development*. London: Adam and Charles Black.

Schweitzer, A. 1955. *Civilization and Ethics*, third edition. London: Adam and Charles Black.

Schweitzer, A. 1966. *My Life and Thought: An Autobiography*. London: Unwin Books.

Selye, H. 1975. *The Stress of Life*, second edition. New York: McGraw-Hill.

Selye, H. 1976. *Stress in Health and Disease*. Boston: Butterworths.

Seruggia, D. and Montoliu, L. 2014. The new CRISPR-Cas system: RNA-guided genome engineering to efficiently produce any desired genetic alteration in animals. *Transgenic Research* 23: 707–716.

Seyfarth, R. M., Cheney, D. L. and Marler, P. 1980. Monkey responses to three different alarm calls: evidence of predator classification and semantic communication. *Science* 210: 801–803.

Shaw, G.B. 1912. *The Uselessness of the Vivisection Inspector*. London: British Union for the Abolition of Vivisection.

Shugg, W. 1968a. Humanitarian attitudes in the early animal experiments of the royal society. *Annals of Science* 24: 227–238.

Shugg, W. 1968b. The Cartesian beast-machine in English literature (1663–1750). *Journal of the History of Ideas* 29: 279–292.

Sikes, R.S. and Bryan, J.A. II. 2015. Institutional animal care and use committee considerations for the use of wildlife in research and education. *ILAR Journal* 56: 335–341.

Sikes, R.S. and the Animal Care and Use Committee of the American Society of Mammalogists 2016. 2016 guidelines of the American Society of Mammalogists for the use of wild mammals in research and education. *Journal of Mammalogy* **97**: 663–688.

Singer, C.J. 1957. *A Short History of Anatomy from the Greeks to Harvey*, second edition. New York: Dover Publications.

Singer, P. 1975. *Animal Liberation*. New York: Avon Books.

Singer, P. 1978. Animal experimentation: philosophical perspectives. In Reich, W.T. (ed.), *Encyclopedia of Bioethics*, Vol. 1, pp. 79–83. New York: Free Press.

Singer, P. 1979. *Practical Ethics*. Cambridge: Cambridge University Press.

Singer, P. 1990. *Animal Liberation*, second edition. London: Jonathan Cape.

Singer, P. 1993. *Practical Ethics*, second edition. Cambridge: Cambridge University Press.

Singer, P. 2011. *Practical Ethics*, third edition. Cambridge: Cambridge University Press.

Singh, P., Schimenti, J.C. and Bolcun-Filas, E. 2015. A mouse geneticist's practical guide to CRISPR applications. *Genetics* **199**: 1–15.

Smith, J.A. and Boyd, K.M. (eds.) 1991. *Lives in the Balance: The Ethics of Using Animals in Biomedical Research*. Oxford: Oxford University Press.

Smyth, D.H. 1978. *Alternatives to Animal Experiments*. London: Scolar Press.

Sneddon, L.U., Elwood, R.W., Adamo, S.A. and Leach, M.C. 2014. Defining and assessing animal pain. *Animal Behaviour* **97**: 201–212.

Stephens, M.L. 1986. *Maternal Deprivation Experiments in Psychology: A Critique of Animal Models*. Jenkinstown, PA: The American Anti-Vivisection Society.

Stephens, M.L. and Mak, N.S. 2014. History of the 3Rs in toxicity testing: from Russell and Burch to 21st century toxicology. In Allen, D.G. and Waters, M.D. (eds.), *Reducing, Refining and Replacing the Use of Animals in Toxicity Testing*, pp. 1–43. Cambridge: The Royal Society of Chemistry.

Stevens, C. 1990. Laboratory animal welfare. In Leavett, E.S. (ed.), *Animals and their Legal Rights*, pp. 66–105. Washington DC: Animal Welfare Institute.

Stone, M. 1989. Cited in *Animal Experimentation, Australian Government, Senate Select Committee on Animal Welfare*. Canberra: Australian Government Publishing Service.

Swami, V., Furnham, A. and Christopher, A.N. 2008. Free the animals? Investigating attitudes toward animal testing in Britain and the United States. *Scandinavian Journal of Psychology* **49**: 269–276.

Tannenbaum, J. and Bennett, B.T. 2015. Russell and Burch's 3Rs then and now: the need for clarity in definition and purpose. *Journal of the American Association for Laboratory Animal Science* **54**: 120–132.

Taylor, K., Gordon, N., Langley, G. and Higgins, W. 2008. Estimates for worldwide laboratory animal use in 2005. *Alternatives to Laboratory Animals* **36**: 327–342.

Townsend, P. and Morton, D.B. 1995. Laboratory animal care policies and regulations: United Kingdom. *ILAR Journal* **37**: 68–74.

Tsunoda, M., Kido, T., Mogi, S., Sugiura, Y., Miyajima, E., Kudo, Y., Kumazawa, T. and Aizawa, Y. 2014. Skin irritation to glass wool or continuous glass filaments as observed by a patch test among human Japanese volunteers. *Industrial Health* **52**: 439–444.

Turner, J. 1980. *Reckoning with the Beast: Animals, Pain and Humanity in the Victorian Mind*. Baltimore, MD: Johns Hopkins University Press.

Tyebkhan, G. 2003. Declaration of Helsinki: the ethical cornerstone of human clinical research. *Indian Journal of Dermatology, Venereology and Leprology* **69**: 245–247.

UK Home Office 2007. *Statistics of Scientific Procedures on Living Animals: Great Britain 2006.* London: The Stationery Office. www.gov.uk/government/statistics/statistics-of-scientific-procedures-on-living-animals-great-britain-2006.

UK Home Office 2014a. *Annual Statistics of Scientific Procedures on Living Animals: Great Britain 2013.* www.gov.uk/government/uploads/system/uploads/attachment_data/file/327854/spanimals13.pdf.

UK Home Office 2014b. *Guidance on the Operation of the Animals (Scientific Procedures) Act 1986.* www.gov.uk/government/uploads/system/uploads/attachment_data/file/291350/Guidance_on_the_Operation_of_ASPA.pdf.

UK Home Office 2015. *The Harm-Benefit Analysis Approach: New Project Licence Applications.* www.gov.uk/government/uploads/system/uploads/attachment_data/file/487914/Harm_Benefit_Analysis__2_.pdf.

UK Home Office 2016. *Annual Statistics of Scientific Procedures on Living Animals: Great Britain 2015.* www.gov.uk/government/uploads/system/uploads/attachment_data/file/537708/scientific-procedures-living-animals-2015.pdf.

United States Department of Agriculture 2013. *Animal Welfare Act and Animal Welfare Regulations.* www.aphis.usda.gov/animal_welfare/downloads/Animal%20Care%20Blue%20Book%20-%202013%20-%20FINAL.pdf.

US Congress, Office of Technology Assessment 1986. *Alternatives to Animal Use in Research, Testing, and Education.* Washington DC: US Government Printing Office.

Use of Fishes in Research Committee 2013. *Guidelines for the Use of Fishes in Research.* Bethesda, MD: American Fisheries Society.

van der Ploeg, A.T. and Reuser, A.J.J. 2008. Pompe's disease. *Lancet* **372**: 1342–1353.

Voltaire, 1764/1962. *Philosophical Dictionary*, pp. 112–113, trans. Gay, P. New York: Basic Books.

Wade, N. 1978. New vaccine may bring man and chimpanzee into tragic conflict. *Science* **200**: 1027–1030.

Wall, P.D. 1992. Humane treatment of animals does not mean treating animals as humans. In Kuchel, T.R., Rose, M. and Burrell, J. (eds.), *Animal Pain: Ethical and Scientific Perspectives*, pp. 1–12. Adelaide: ACCART.

Walsh, M. and Richmond, J. 2005. Regulation of animal experimentation in the United Kingdom. *School Science Review* **87** (319): 85–89.

Waugh, C. and Monamy, V. 2016. Opposing lethal wildlife research when non-lethal methods exist: scientific whaling as a case study. *Journal of Fish and Wildlife Management* **7**: 231–236.

Weiss, J.M. 1972. Psychological factors in stress and disease. *Scientific American* **226**: 104–113.

Wells, D.J., Playle, L.C., Enser, W.E., Flecknell, P.A., Gardiner, M.A., Holland, J., Howard, B.R., Hubrecht, R., Humphreys, K.R., Jackson, I.J., Lane, N., Maconochie, M., Mason, G., Morton, D.B., Raymond, R., Robinson, V., Smith, J.A. and Watt, N. 2006. Assessing the welfare of genetically altered mice. *Laboratory Animals* **40**: 111–114.

White, J.R. 2014. A brief history of the development of diabetes medications. *Diabetes Spectrum* **27**: 82–86.

Whittaker, A.L. and Howarth, G.S. 2014. Use of spontaneous behaviour measures to assess pain in laboratory rats and mice: how are we progressing? *Applied Animal Behaviour Science* **151**: 1–12.

Wick, P. Chortarea, S., Guenat, O.T., Roesslein, M., Stucki, J.D., Hirn, S., Petri-Fink, A. and Rothen-Rutishauser, B. 2015. *In vitro-ex vivo* model systems for nanosafety assessment. *European Journal of Nanomedicine* **7**: 169–179.

Wickens, S.M. 2007. *Science in the Service of Animal Welfare: A Chronicle of Eighty Years of Service*. London: UFAW.

Wise, S.M. 2000. *Rattling the Cage: Towards Legal Rights for Animals*. Cambridge, MA: Perseus Books.

Wise, S.M. 2002. *Drawing the Line: Science and the Case for Animal Rights*. Cambridge, MA: Perseus Books.

Wolfensohn, S. and Lloyd, M. 2013. *Handbook of Laboratory Animal Management and Welfare*, fourth edition. Oxford: Wiley-Blackwell.

Wong, J. 1995. Laboratory animal care policies and regulations: Canada. *ILAR Journal* 37: 57–59.

World Health Organisation. 2015. *Global Health Observatory Data*. www.who.int/gho/ mortality_burden_disease/life_tables/situation_trends/en/.

Yum, S., Woo, S., Lee, A., Won, H. and Kim, J. 2014. *Hydra*, a candidate for an alternative model in environmental genomics. *Molecular and Cellular Toxicology* 10: 339–346.

Zhang, J., Hsieh, J. and Zhu, H. 2014. Profiling animal toxicants by automatically mining public bioassay data: a big data approach for computational toxicology. *PloS One* 9(6): e99863. doi: 10.1371/journal.pone.0099863.

Zheng, F., Fu, F., Cheng, Y., Wang, C., Zhao, Y. and Gu, Z. 2016. Organ-on-a-chip systems: microengineering to biomimic living systems. *Small* 12: 2253–2282.

Zhu, H., Kim, M., Zhang, L. and Sedykh, A. 2014. Computers instead of cells: computational modelling of chemical toxicity. In Allen, D.G. and Waters, M.D. (eds.), *Reducing, Refining and Replacing the Use of Animals in Toxicity Testing*, pp. 163–182. Cambridge: The Royal Society of Chemistry.

# Index